GOUT DIET

The Purine Myth

by

Rose Scott

The Food That Really Causes Gout

COPYRIGHT

Gout Diet: The Purine Myth

First Edition

Copyright Rose Scott 2014.

The moral right of the author has been asserted.

All rights reserved. No part of this publication may be reproduced , stored in a retrieval system or transmitted in any form or by any means without the prior permission of the copyright owner.

ISBN - 13: 978-1502509178
ISBN - 10: 1502509172

DISCLAIMER

This book provides general information only. It is based on information gathered from a large number of different sources. It does not provide any form of medical advice and it is not a substitute for the advice of your own doctor, medical practitioner or health care professional. Readers are specifically advised to consult their doctor regarding the treatment of any medical condition that they have. The author of this book shall not be held liable or responsible for any misuse or misunderstanding of the information contained in this book or for any loss, damage or injury caused or alleged to be caused either directly or indirectly by any action that is consequential to reading the contents of this book.
No part of this book has been evaluated or approved by any medical, scientific, professional or Food or Drug Administration Authority

CONTENTS

INTRODUCTION

Is Gout A Wakeup Call?

Gout has afflicted man for thousands of years. It is one of the most painful and debilitating diseases and it affects millions of people around the world. It leaves them facing a lifetime of pain.

If you have ever asked the question *"Why do I have gout"?* you will almost invariably have been told that it is because you have too much uric acid, something which is bound to be your fault as it is caused by eating too much purine rich food and drinking too much alcohol. The solution, drugs to reduce the amount of uric acid and a low purine diet. Notwithstanding that a rigid purine restricted diet is well nigh impossible to sustain for long, it is a diet that is based on miss-information and not facts. It is also high in the refined carbohydrates that actually cause gout and low in the Omega-3 essential fatty acids that your body desperately needs to enable it to fight the inflammation that gout causes At the end of the day a low purine diet will simply make things worse.

Nature has given us some simple and straightforward ways of keeping ourselves healthy. For years we have been told that uric acid serves no biological purpose and that our bodies do not need it. Absolutely not true. Uric acid is an important antioxidant and it is also a marker of tissue injury that acts as one of the regulators of our immune system. Uric acid helps our bodies deal with trauma. So when our body is under assault and confronted by an imbalance of free radicals and damaged cells, irrespective of where these come from, our body's antioxidant defences and our immune system swing into action in order to put things right. Uric acid levels increase and Oxidative Stress develops. High levels of uric acid are a warning sign that things are going wrong. They are a sign that our body is out of balance and under stress and that it is calling out for help.

We need a major re-think of how we look at high levels of uric acid and gout. Uric acid is not the bad guy it is made out to be. Rather than using drugs to get rid of the uric acid, a more holistic approach is to find out what is causing the stress and trauma our body is being subjected to and then eliminate the problems. That way we have a chance of getting the body back in balance and functioning normally.

Gout Diet The Purine Myth is all about understanding what we need to do to get our body back into working order. Five years ago my husband was crippled by gout. Today he lives a gout free life. I sincerely hope that this book will give you the knowledge and motivation you need to take control of your health and take the first steps towards leading a gout free life.

What Causes Gout?

Gout has afflicted mankind for thousands of years. Today it is the most common form of inflammatory arthritis found in industrialised countries. In what is loosely described as the 'Western World', between 1% and 2% of men in their 50's and up to 7% of men in their 70's now suffer from gout. While hither too it was mainly a male disease women, particularly post menopausal women, are now being increasingly afflicted. Why is gout increasing so rapidly? Possible explanations include lifestyle, high levels of pollution, the overall ageing of the population and changes to our diet made possible by increased prosperity and new food manufacturing processes. In reality we just do not know.

Of all of the forms of arthritis gout is the one we understand the best. Yet despite this the actual "cause" of gout still remains somewhat obscure. Over the years medical science has studied it in great detail and correlated its occurrence to both diet and lifestyle. In the process it has gained a good understanding of how it affects the body, but with the development of Allopurinol and other drugs such as Probenecid interest in finding out what actually causes gout diminished. Gout became a 'treatable' disease and, as is so often the case, the 'cure' became more important than understanding the cause and preventing the onset of the disease in the first place. However, as the treatment of gout is often poorly managed and only around 40% of the medications prescribed are actually effective, there is still a real need to understand more about the disease.

What we do know is that gout is all to do with uric acid, a weak organic acid that occurs naturally in your blood, and the crystals that it sometimes forms. If you suffer from gout you are likely to have a higher than 'normal' amount of uric acid in your blood, in medical terms you suffer from Hyperuricemia, and because uric acid is not very soluble, microscopic crystals have formed and accumulated in the soft tissue in one or some of your joints. Most commonly a big toe or an ankle is the target but any joint can be affected. Your body sees these crystals as 'foreign bodies' and your immune system responds accordingly, sending out antibodies to fight them off. Hence the inflammation and from this the excruciating pain.

If you have an "above normal" amount of uric acid is it inevitable that you will develop gout? Not necessarily. Strangely only between 10% and 20% of people with hyperuricemia actually develop gout. What is known for sure though is that for most people, once crystals of uric acid have formed, gout 'flares' or attacks will recur over and over again, usually at increasingly frequent intervals.

Men naturally have higher levels of uric acid than women and as a consequence an increased prevalence of gout. This however becomes less pronounced as we get older. Why the difference between men and women? Well it may be explained in women of childbearing age by the presence of oestrogen, which is known to have the effect of making the kidneys more efficient at removing uric acid. As a consequence gout is rare in young women. However, post menopause as oestrogen levels fall, uric acid levels increase and gout becomes more prevalent. By the time they reach their 70's women are just as likely to develop gout as men.

Uric Acid

Uric acid is formed inside our bodies when organic compounds called purines are broken down or in biochemical terminology 'catabolised'. Because of this purines are often said to be the bane of the gout sufferers life and for years we have been told to avoid them or to reduce their intake. Because of their association with gout purines have acquired a reputation of being in some way 'bad'. Yet nothing could be farther from the truth. They are in fact one of the building blocks of all living organisms on earth. Everything from simple viruses to complex multi-cellular creatures contain them. As such they are among the most important of all biological molecules. Without them our chromosomes and the genetic material in all living creatures would simply not exist.

For many years uric acid was considered to be an inert waste product that, when present in higher than normal levels, was known for the harmful and troublesome effects of causing gout and kidney stones. Even now many sources of information on gout tell you that *"uric acid serves no biological or biochemical function"*. However, we now know much more about uric acid and it's various functions and beneficial effects and one of these is that it is a powerful antioxidant. In fact uric acid has the highest concentration of any of the water soluble antioxidants found in our blood and it provides nearly half its antioxidant capacity. Surprisingly the antioxidant properties of uric acid are fifty times as powerful as those of Vitamin C. Is uric acid the only antioxidant our body makes? No, it is just one of a sophisticated team of antioxidants that our bodies make in order to protect itself from free radicals and repair the damage that free radicals cause.

The scientific community has known about uric acid's function as an antioxidant since 1981. But despite this it is something that is seldom mentioned. When you read about gout, uric acid is invariably depicted as being 'bad', a sort of villain that only causes trouble. This is clearly not the case. Our bodies need uric acid, in fact without it they would simply not function properly.

How are purines converted into uric acid? As with all metabolic processes enzymes are needed and in the case of uric acid the last one in a long multi-stage process is an enzyme called Xanthine Oxidase. If you have too little Xanthine Oxidase you don't make enough uric acid and if you have too much you have the potential to make too much uric acid. The drug Allopurinol that is used to treat gout inhibits the way Xanthine Oxidase works and as a consequence it reduces the amount of uric acid the body is able to produce.

The relationship between uric acid and the human body is complex and many questions about the part it plays have yet to be answered. One thing is certain however, the human body needs uric acid. It is an essential part of our body's biochemistry and it plays a major role not only in its antioxidant defences but also in inflammation and our immune response.

Inflammation & Our Immune Response

Inflammation is a topic that is attracting a lot of attention at the moment as it appears to be associated with many of the chronic diseases that are afflicting the Western World. Gout is a form of inflammatory arthritis, so if you have gout parts of your body are in a state of inflammation. Because of this understanding inflammation and how it affects your body is important.

The word inflammation comes from the Latin word *'inflammo'* meaning *'I set alight, I ignite'*. When something harmful or irritating affects a part of your body there is an automatic response to try to remove it. When you catch a cold or sprain your ankle your immune system moves into gear and triggers a chain of events that is referred to as the inflammatory cascade. The familiar signs of inflammation, raised temperature, localised heat, pain, swelling and redness, are the first signs that your immune system is being called into action and they show you that your body is trying to heal itself.

Inflammation is part of the body's 'innate' immune response, something that is present even before we are born. Innate immunity is an automatic immunity that is not directed towards anything specific. As we go through life and are exposed to diseases or vaccinated against them we acquire 'adaptive' immunity. In a delicate balance of give-and-take inflammation begins when 'pro-inflammatory hormones' in your body call out for your white blood cells to come and clear out an infection or repair damaged tissue. These pro-inflammatory hormones are matched by equally powerful closely related 'anti-inflammatory' compounds which move in once the threat is neutralised to begin the healing process.

The inflammation we experience during our daily lives can be either 'acute' or 'chronic'. Chronic inflammation is sometimes referred to as 'systemic' inflammation. Acute inflammation that ebbs and flows as needed signifies a well balanced immune system. Colds, flu and childhood diseases mean that inflammation and a rise in temperature starts suddenly and quickly progresses to become severe. The signs and symptoms are only present for a few days and they soon subside. On occasion in cases of severe illness they can last for a few weeks but this is unusual.

Sometimes, however, as in the case of chronic or systemic inflammation, the inflammation itself can cause further inflammation. It can become self perpetuating and sometimes last for months or even years. Symptoms of inflammation that do not go away are telling you that the switch to your immune system is stuck in the 'on' position. It is poised on high alert and is unable to shut itself off. Some people believe that chronic irritants, food sensitivities and common allergens like the proteins found in dairy products and wheat can trigger this type of chronic inflammation. It is now a widely accepted fact that the food we eat can be either 'pro' or 'anti' inflammatory.

The study of inflammation and our immune system is a relatively new science. While there is still an enormous amount to learn there is no doubt that the human immune response is an extremely sophisticated finely balanced mechanism. Without it we would not be able to survive the most minor infection or the tiniest cut. Some scientists believe that like other things in our evolutionary history this sophisticated immune response gave our early ancestors a major survival advantage. As with so much about the human body how such a sophisticated response came about is unclear. It is certainly the subject of a great deal of speculation.

Inflammation occurs when tissues in our body are damaged or when we are 'attacked' by bacteria or viruses. Substances like pro inflammatory hormones are produced by our body and these alert it to the danger and tell our immune system to switch itself on. Uric acid behaves like one of these pro inflammatory hormones. It is not involved in our immune response to bacteria and viruses but it is involved when our bodies are subjected to trauma and when cells are damaged or die. The large amounts of uric acid that are produced in the immediate vicinity of damaged, dying or dead cells stimulates a type of immune cell called dendritic cells to mature and swing into action. Effectively uric acid has a sort of immune boosting effect and it plays a fundamental part in protecting our bodies from tissue damage and trauma.

In the Western World chronic or systemic inflammation is on the rise. We know this from inflammatory markers and the pro inflammatory and anti inflammatory hormones that our body's produce. Most degenerative diseases involve an element of chronic low level inflammation and the inability to turn off important inflammatory processes when they are no longer needed. Gout is one of these diseases.

Can Food Cause Inflammation?

When our bodies metabolise the food we eat some of the nutrients in it are used to produce substances called prostaglandins. These prostaglandins are a sort of chemical messenger and they can be either pro-inflammatory, in other words they create inflammation or increase a state of inflammation that already exists, or they can be anti-inflammatory and calm down or reduce inflammation. Imbalances in your diet can lead to excessive amounts of inflammatory prostaglandins being produced.

If you suffer from gout your body is in a state of chronic systemic inflammation. Any pro inflammatory food you consume will simply fuel this inflammation. Refined grains, animal products, processed meats, sugar, polyunsaturated vegetable oils, hydrogenated oils in the form of trans fats, 'regular' soft drinks and foods that are fried and cooked at high temperatures, are on most people's menus and these are all inflammatory. In contrast anti-inflammatory foods like wholegrains, beans and pulses, nuts and seeds, fresh fruit and vegetables, herbs and spices and oily fish form a very small part of a typical Western diet.

Probably the two most important foods that are fuelling inflammation are polyunsaturated vegetable oils and sugar, in all their forms and disguises. Iron rich foods come in a close third. Notwithstanding that the consumption of sugar has increased enormously over the last hundred years, it is the polyunsaturated vegetable oils that are the most interesting as they are effectively a new kid on the block and its a pretty unruly kid at that.

"Your Body is Too Acidic "

How many times have you read that if you suffer from gout it is because your body and your blood is "too acidic". It is true you almost certainly have a higher than normal level of uric acid but your body and blood is most definitely not "too acidic". If it was you would be suffering from acidosis and you would be either extremely ill or dead!

At all times the human body needs to be slightly alkaline and it works very hard to keep itself that way. When you eat and drink the end products of digestion and the assimilation of the nutrients in the food and drink results in either an overall acid or alkaline effect on your body. Because our body needs to be slightly alkaline, it uses its natural buffer systems to regulate its acidity and alkalinity. Under normal circumstances this works fine but if you spend years eating a diet that is highly acidic these buffers ultimately become exhausted and the body has to call on its reserves, in particular something called its calcium phosphate reserves. When this happens it heads in the direction of our bones, joints and teeth and takes small amounts of calcium phosphate from them. This is where there is a link between the consumption of 'acidic' foods and gout.

In the process of calling on and using these calcium phosphate reserves the concentration of minute particles of calcium in the form of ions in the blood increases slightly and this increases the risk of crystals of uric acid 'seeding' around the ions and triggering an attack of gout. A similar process can happen when there are sudden short term 'spikes' in the acidity of our blood due to a build up of lactic acid. Something that can result from extreme exercise, sleep apnoea or the excessive consumption of alcohol.

So which foods have an alkaline forming effect and which have an acid forming effect? Well most wheat grains, animal products, sugar, alcohol and highly processed foods have an acid forming effect and generally speaking most vegetables, fruit and unprocessed foods have an alkaline forming effect. Compared to vegetarians, people who eat animal protein, particularly in the form of meat, lose between two and four times the amount of calcium. The larger the amount of animal protein consumed and the longer the length of time over which it is consumed, the greater the loss of calcium.

Unfortunately vegetables, fruit and unprocessed foods are in short supply in the typical Western diet. Ideally you need to eat slightly more alkaline forming foods than acid forming foods in order to reduce the pressure on your body's buffer systems.

Free Radicals Antioxidants & Oxidative Stress

Free Radicals

The majority of life forms that exist on earth need oxygen to live, yet one of the paradoxes of this is that oxygen is a highly reactive molecule that can damage living organisms by producing free radicals. Heard of Free Radicals but not sure what they are? Put simply, a Free Radical is an atom, molecule of part of an atom called an ion that is 'unstable'. This instability is due to its structure. If it has one or more unpaired electrons it is known as a Free Radical. Because they are unstable, Free Radicals try to make themselves stable by 'stealing' electrons from other atoms, molecules or ions and the process of doing this they often cause damage.

Simply by living and deriving energy from the air we breathe and the food we eat our bodies produce Free Radicals. Many of these are needed in controlled amounts to maintain life and keep us in good health, others however can react with cells, fats and proteins inside our bodies and cause damage. Free radicals are all around us. We breath them in from cigarette smoke, car exhausts and air pollution, the ultra violet rays from the sun create them when we are exposed to sunlight and we consume them in our food and sometimes the water we drink.

An imbalance or overload of Free Radicals can impair our immune system and it is a potential factor in many modern day illnesses. In order for us to be able to lead healthy lives the Free Radicals need to be neutralised and rendered harmless. In order to do this we need antioxidants.

Antioxidants

Antioxidants are stable molecules that have 'spare' electrons. They are able to neutralise Free Radicals by sacrificing these spare electrons. This effectively makes the Free Radicals safe.

The human body has a complex internally produced team of antioxidants that it uses to defend itself from Free Radicals, In addition the food we eat also provides us with antioxidants; Vitamin C (ascorbate), Vitamin E and the beta carotenes are just some of the 8,000 antioxidants that nature provides. Some antioxidants work as a team and can interact with other antioxidants to regenerate their original properties once they have been used.

Oxidative Stress

The more Free Radicals we are exposed to the more antioxidants our body needs to keep them in check. Under normal balanced conditions Free Radicals are rendered harmless either by our body's own antioxidants or by the antioxidants we consume in our food. However, if we are not consuming enough antioxidants or enough of the raw materials or 'building blocks' that our body needs to make its own antioxidants, the damaging effect of the Free Radicals remains unchecked. Our antioxidant defences are overwhelmed and the antioxidant to pro-oxidant balance shifts in favour of the Free Radicals. Damage to the body occurs and a state of Oxidative Stress develops.

The Free Radicals that are left unchecked damage cells and other components of the cells. A cell is able to overcome small amounts of damage and regain its original state, but severe Oxidative Stress can have toxic effects that can result in trauma and widespread cell death. When this happens uric acid is produced in the immediate vicinity of the dying or dead cells in order to stimulate the immune response and the inflammatory cascade begins. The scale of the Oxidative Stress, the amount of uric acid that is generated and the level of inflammation that this causes depends entirely on the degree of the imbalance between the Free Radicals and the antioxidants.

Its all about balance

The breakdown of purines and their conversion into uric acid is a major source of free radicals. These are produced in the form of 'Superoxide'. Under normal healthy balanced conditions these superoxides are rendered harmless by one of the body's own antioxidants, Superoxide Dismutase (SOD). However, if conditions are not balanced and for some reason the body is unable to supply enough Superoxide Dismutase, the excess superoxide generated acts as a free radical and ultimately ends up contributing to and increasing the state of oxidative stress in the body. This in turn leads to the influx of inflammatory cells and general state of inflammation that can trigger the onset of many chronic diseases.

Why do Uric Acid Levels Rise?

Hyperuricemia, a higher than normal level of uric acid, is thought to result from either the over production of uric acid or the under excretion of uric acid. On occasion it can be a combination of both. Above normal amounts of uric acid can also be a primary or secondary result of a medical condition or the use of certain types of drugs and medication. The general consensus appears to be that the over production of uric acid accounts for 10% of the cause of hyperuricemia and the under excretion of uric acid for 90%.

Clearly Oxidative Stress can lead to increased levels of uric acid and this means that when the body is in a state of Oxidative Stress it needs to excrete more than the 'normal' amount of uric acid if uric acid levels are to be maintained at a 'normal' level. This inevitably increases the pressure on the bodies removal and excretion processes. Sugar in the form of fructose is known to directly increase levels of uric acid but if 'over production' is only 10% of the problem what prevents us from excreting uric acid and keeping our body in balance?

Well there are quite a lot of reasons. Insulin Resistance and diabetes play a significant part as high levels of insulin are known to increase the amount of uric acid that is reabsorbed after it has been filtered out by the kidneys. This directly reduces the amount of uric acid that is excreted. Fructose scores twice because as well as directly increasing levels of uric acid it also prevents us excreting it effectively. Lifestyle and genetics both affect the way our bodies remove uric acid but age is also a major factor.

We know that the incidence of gout and hyperuricemia increases with age and there are many reasons for this. Not least is that as we get older our bodies do not function quite as well as they used to; our kidneys aren't as efficient as they used to be at excreting waste products and our pancreas isn't as efficient as it used to be at regulating the production of insulin. In addition the natural turnover of cells in our bodies increases as we get older and as these cells become damaged and die they increase the load of uric acid that the body has to handle.

With time we all age, some faster then others. In 1956 a "free radical theory of ageing" was proposed and over the years this has gained wide acceptance. It is a fact that the body's production of free radicals and the damage free radicals cause increases with age. However, scientists have now identified something that they believe speeds up the ageing process. Advanced Glycation End products, also known as AGE's or Glycotoxins, are relatively new players on the health and nutrition scene but they are now considered to be one of the primary factors in ageing and degenerative diseases. Not only do they damage cells and encourage inflammation and oxidative stress, they are also strongly associated with degenerative diseases like diabetes and reduced kidney function, all of which impair the way in which the kidneys work and excrete uric acid.

When our bodies breakdown purines into uric acid it uses an enzyme called Xanthine Oxidase. We know that gout is more common in men than women and one of the reasons for this is the male sex hormone testosterone. As we get older we tend to accumulate iron, so the amount of iron in the body increases with age, especially in men, as the amount of iron in women of childbearing age is regulated by their menstrual cycle. Readily available iron activates Xanthine Oxidase and another trace element in our bodies, copper, deactivates it. So copper effectively puts a sort of 'brake' on Xanthine Oxidase and our ability to produce uric acid. Testosterone increases the half life of copper. In other words the copper is more effective and stays effective for longer when there is testosterone around. For most men while they are young, things are in balance. However, as men age and the AGE's mentioned earlier can accelerate the ageing process, their levels of testosterone fall and because the 'life' of the available copper reduces the brake the copper puts on the Xanthine Oxidase also reduces. The Xanthine Oxidase becomes more active and this results in the potential for the body to make much more uric acid.

The Purine Myth

Uric Acid is formed when purines are broken down and metabolised but where do the purines come from?

Well, food is one source of purines but our own bodies also provide a source of purines when our cells die, either through the natural process of 'programmed' cell death or Apoptosis, or because cells become damaged by free radicals and other damage causing agents. The amount of purine coming from our own body is surprisingly high. Some scientists say that 70% of the purines our body uses come from ourselves (endogenous purines) and 30% from our food (exogenous purines), others that up to 90% come from our bodies and only 10% from our food. Clearly if the body is under stress and traumatised and as a consequence cells die or become damaged and need to be replaced in higher than normal numbers, the ratio between the purines we eat and the purines our bodies produce will change.

For years science and the medical profession have told us that purines cause gout and that a low purine diet will cure it. Books, learned journals and web sites are still telling us the same thing. The general consensus is that over production of uric acid accounts for 10% of the cause of hyperuricemia and the under excretion of uric acid for 90%. On the assumption that these figures are correct the conventional 'low purine' diet that is recommended for gout does not hold up. A low purine diet only addresses the 10% issue of the over production of uric acid not the 90% under excretion. If 70% of the purines for this over production come from our body's own turnover of cells, the purines we obtain from our food would contribute at best only one third of this 10%, a very small amount.

In view of this, logic says that the "excessive intake of dietary purines" can rarely if ever be the cause of the over production of uric acid and gout. Interestingly as long ago as 1984 a scientist called Irvine Fox, who studied gout in great detail, noted that a low purine diet was ineffective and had only a minor effect on gout.

In reality a low purine diet is well nigh impossible to follow and it is probably one of the worse possible diets for gout. Not only is it imbalanced, it is also high in carbohydrates and if you suffer from gout a large amount of carbohydrate is one thing your body most definitely does not need.

How did the purine myth come about?

Red meat, especially organ meat, contains high levels of purines and purines are the building blocks from which uric acid is made. As a consequence for centuries the consumption of red meat has been linked to gout. From an epidemiological perspective the link between meat, poultry and fish consumption and gout is inevitable as animal products are a major component of a "Western diet". However, this diet is also high in sugar, refined carbohydrates, processed foods and vegetable oils and it is extremely low in fresh fruit and vegetables. As a consequence despite everyone's best efforts it is almost impossible to separate the consumption of meat from the consumption of the other foods and prove any direct cause and effect relationships. However, as you will read later, when you look at the impact iron can have on the development of gout and then look at the sources of iron in our diet it is clear that there is an undeniable link between hyperuricemia, gout and the consumption of animal products. Somewhat ironically and contrary to conventional dietary advice, this is not because of the purines that these animal products contain, it is the iron.

In reality purines are innocent by-standers that have been historically been given a bad press. They are simply the raw material our body uses to make uric acid. Why our body needs to increase the amount of uric acid it makes and hang on to the uric acid that it has made is the key issue in understanding what causes gout.

WHERE DID IT ALL GO WRONG?

In less than 100 years the general state of health of the western world has deteriorated rapidly and it is continuing to do so at an alarming rate. In 1980 150 million people were thought to be suffering from diabetes. Today this figure is nearer to 360 million. Even among children metabolic syndrome and obesity is close to becoming an epidemic. When it comes to gout things are even worse. A long term study that was recently published in the UK showed that the prevalence of gout rose by 64% during the course of the 15 year study, an astounding increase of around 4% a year.

If we look back into even recent history it is clear that both our lifestyle and our diet have changed dramatically. Lack of exercise, junk food and TV diners are all taking their toll on our health. Whether we like it or not, the bottom line is that we all eat too much. We simply eat more than our bodies need and most of us are unaware that we are doing this because large amounts of sugar and the wrong sort of fat are hidden in our food. We are also eating too much of the wrong foods. Foods that are actually damaging our health. We have been fed misinformation and in effect conned by big business and advertising into believing that some foods are good for us when in fact they are not. The triumph of partially hydrogenated vegetable fats in the form of margarine and low fat spreads as being a healthier option than butter is a classical example of this.

So where did it go wrong? We all lead busy lives and as a consequence quick meals are sometimes a necessity. For most of us cooking and preparing food is seen as a chore. Many of us would prefer to watch TV or read a book than cook. The problem really started when we began to 'manufacture' food, and I mean 'manufacture' in the widest sense of the word. The intensive farming of beef and poultry is just another type of manufacturing. When we started manufacturing food it became available in large quantities at a price that ordinary people could afford. At the same time it became easy for us to eat food that would otherwise take a long time to prepare and cook. Luxury foods like biscuits, cookies, cakes, chips, fries, mayonnaise and processed meats became widely available, so the ordinary man was able to eat more and at the same time also adopt some of the eating habits of the rich. Sixty years ago you were lucky if you ate meat once a week. Now many people eat it every day, sometimes at every meal. How often do you eat chicken or turkey? Well sixty years ago chicken and turkey were luxury foods. They were the preserve of the wealthy. The ordinary man was lucky if he ate them once a year at Christmas or Thanksgiving, now we can eat them any time we want.

In the early 1920's average uric acid levels across the American population were around 3.5 mg/dl. In the past 90 years they have risen to between 4.0 and 5.5mg/dl. An enormous increase that brings the 'average' close to the 'above normal' level. How many 'manufactured' foods were available in 1920? Nowhere near the number there are today. When did they first appear on the scene? Well we know that sugar goes back a very long way. But what about breakfast cereals. They were first packaged as a wholegrain health food in the late 1800's, but by the 1920's they began to evolve into the sugar coated flakes, hoops and puffs that we know today.

Why did we change our eating habits and adopt manufactured and processed foods as part of our daily diet so quickly? The answer to this would fill volumes. What we do know is that many of the manufactured foods that have come onto the scene since the early 1900's are a smoking gun when it comes to gout and other chronic diseases. Vegetable oils, trans fats, over refined carbohydrates, sugar and processed meats are most certainly not contributing positively to the health of the nation.

When it comes to the food industry, it is very difficult not to become political. However, it is an undeniable fact that food manufacturing is now big business, with companies spending billions of dollars a year on aggressive advertising that is geared to preserving their bottom line profits and not the health and well being of the people consuming the food they make.

Manufactured foods bring with them a whole raft of problems not least of which is the addition of compounds that are designed to enhance their appearance and extend their shelf life. Most food processing takes out many of the good things and adds back in a lot of bad things. Manufactured and processed foods are generally speaking impoverished products. Because of this our diet contains too many calories that have been stripped of most of the essential trace nutrients necessary for their proper assimilation. The high-speed milling of grains such as wheat, rice, and corn results in the reduction or removal of more than twenty nutrients, including some essential fatty acids and the majority of their minerals and trace elements. In order to make your body's internally produced antioxidant team you need these minerals and trace elements. Without these antioxidants free radicals are not neutralised and oxidative stress develops at an ever-increasing rate.

Like many things in life food can be addictive and manufactured and processed foods really are addictive, the food manufacturers have made sure of that. Dietary habits are just that, habits, and like all habits they can be changed. However, urging someone to change the eating habits of a lifetime is no easy task. It is a fact that less than 20% of patients seeking medical advice are prepared to make substantial lifestyle and dietary changes. In the management of gout, dietary and lifestyle changes are crucially important. If you suffer from gout your body is not functioning properly, in fact it is crying out for help. In order to get it back into proper working order, the essential first step towards leading a gout free life, you need a long term solution. There is no magic cure or silver bullet.

For years the gout sufferer has been told that cherry juice, apple cider vinegar, bicarbonate of soda, red cabbage, tablets of green tea and special food supplements are wonder foods that will cure their gout. The sad reality is that you cannot rectify a diet that is overloaded with the wrong foods and completely lacking in the essential vitamins, minerals and antioxidants it so desperately needs by simply taking a one off cure. We need to look at the 'big picture' and correct the underlying causes of gout and surprisingly this is some of the food that many of us we eat on an almost daily basis.

- Polyunsaturated Vegetable Oils and Trans Fats
- Food that contains iron
- Refined Carbohydrates
- Sugar and High Fructose Corn Syrup
- Fruit juice and smoothies.
- Cooking Methods that fry, grill and roast at high temperatures
- Alcohol; Beer, Lager, Cider, Wine and Spirits

If you are reading this you are one of the 20% of gout sufferers who are prepared to make, or at least think about making some changes to your diet and lifestyle. The purpose of the next section of this book is to provide you with the information that will help you make these changes.

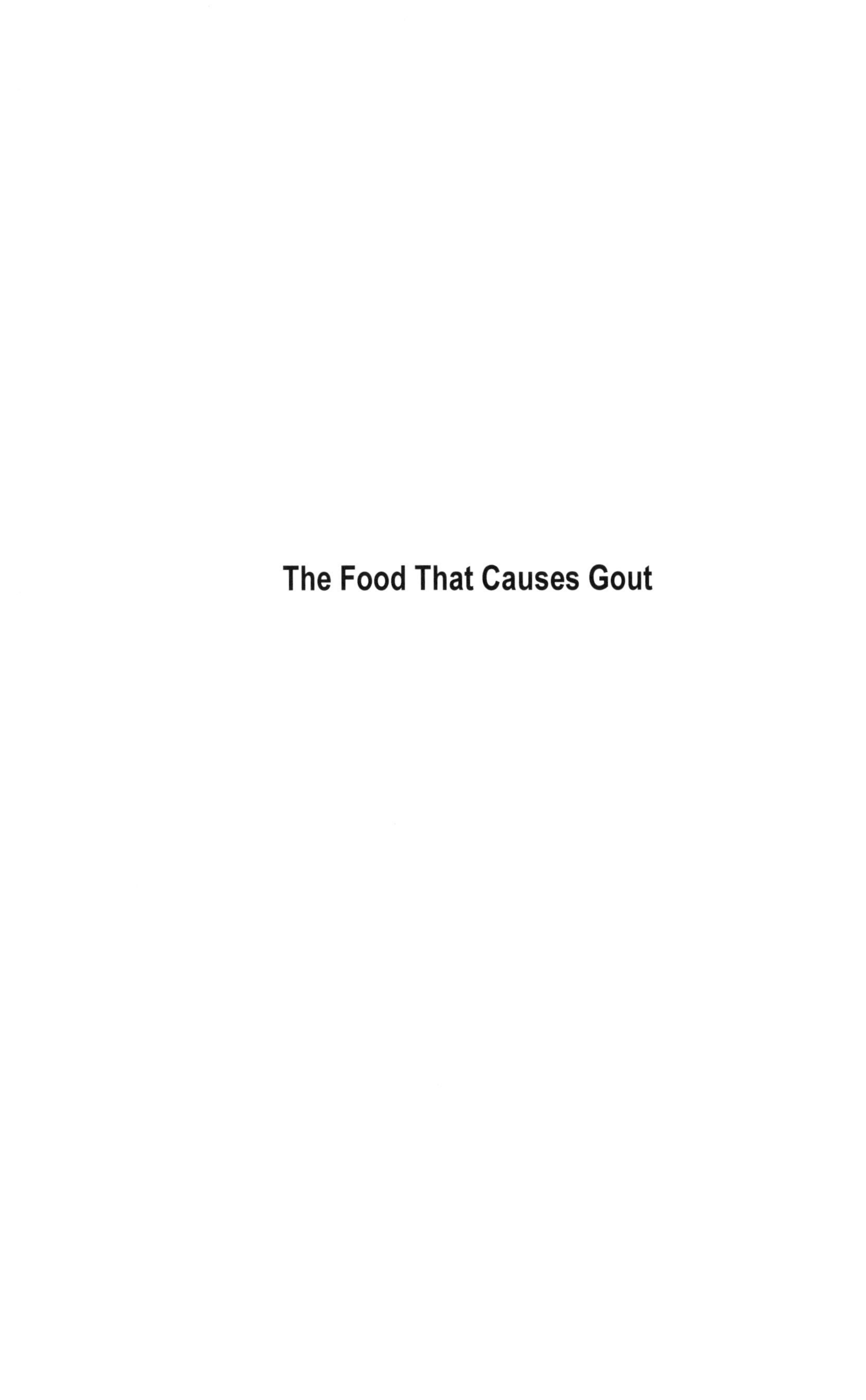

The Food That Causes Gout

VEGETABLE OILS & "TRANS FATS"

Sunflower, safflower, rapeseed, canola, peanut (ground nut or arachnide) and soya oils as well as margarines, "low fat" and "lite" spreads but most definitely not olive oil. Olive oil is one of the "good guys"

If you asked the question which is worse for your health, white flour, sugar or vegetable oils, most people would answer white flour or sugar. But are they really the bad guys they are made out to be? They have both been around for quite a while. Just look at some Victorian and Edwardian cookbooks. People ate them then and they were generally far healthier than we are today. In reality white flour and sugar are not fundamentally bad. What is bad is the enormous amounts of them that we are now consuming. Polyunsaturated vegetable oils on the other hand are something that did not exist a hundred years ago. They are entirely new and entirely unnatural foods that have crept stealthily into our diets. Because of the damage they can cause, they are being described by some as the "health villains" of the 20th Century.

Why are Polyunsaturated Vegetable Oils bad for us?

Put simply our bodies are unable to handle them, especially in the amounts we are currently consuming them in. Our bodies need polyunsaturated vegetable oils but only in very small quantities. For almost all human history they have been consumed only in the small amounts that occur naturally in nuts and seeds, and nuts and seeds are complex foods that contain many other nutrients as well as the polyunsaturated vegetable oils. It is only since industrialised extraction processes came onto the scene that we have eaten them in large quantities. In order to understand why polyunsaturated vegetable oils are so bad we first need to understand what they are and where they fit into the big picture of fats and oils.

Fats and Oils

The technical or scientific name for fats and vegetable oils is 'fatty acids'. 'Lipids' is the medical name that is used to describe them. They are a class of organic substances that are not soluble in water. In simple terms they are made from chains of carbon and hydrogen atoms that are 'bound' together in different ways and held together at one end by a sort of "head' that is made from carbon and oxygen atoms. The chains come in different lengths, they are twisted together and 'bent' in different ways and they come with different degrees of 'saturation'. A fat is 'saturated' when all of the available atoms of carbon and hydrogen are linked together and this makes them very stable. Because they are stable they do not oxidise or in technical terms become 'rancid' even when they are heated for cooking purposes. As a general rule the more saturated a fat is the more stable it is and the more beneficial and safer it is to eat.

Fats and oils can be divided into three groups:-

- **Saturated fats:** These have no free atoms of hydrogen, do not oxidise easily and are solid at room temperature.
- **Monounsaturated fats:** These have two hydrogen atoms missing and are usually liquid at room temperature. Like saturated fats they are relatively stable and do not oxidise or go rancid easily.
- **Polyunsaturated fats:** These have four or more hydrogen atoms missing and are liquid even when cold. These oils are very unstable and highly reactive. Even in their natural state they oxidise and go rancid easily and this is why nature has packaged them up neatly inside nuts and seeds with their own supply of antioxidants and vitamins to protect them. As a consequence once they are extracted they become chemically highly reactive and they contain a lot of free radicals.

Polyunsaturated fats and oils are referred to as PUFA's. They are found in different amounts in all natural foods including meat, fish, vegetables and seeds. In general, vegetable oils such as sunflower, safflower, corn, soy, flax seed, sesame seed, pumpkin seed and canola or rapeseed oils are the most concentrated sources of PUFA's in our diet. These oils contain different types of fats in different proportions and they are broadly classified into 4 groups; Omega 3, Omega 6, Omega 9 and Conjugated fatty acids. Some, like Omega-3 and Omega-6, are essential for our body to work properly. As our body is unable to make these fats they are called "essential" fatty acids or EFA's and these need to be obtained from the food we eat.

Essential Fatty Acids or EFA's

Most of us have heard about essential fatty acids, the names Omega-3 and Omega-6 usually come to mind. But what exactly are they and why are they so important?

The Omega 3 and Omega 6 groups of fatty acids each contain a number of different fatty acids, most of which the body is either able to make or obtain directly from food. In order to make fatty acid in the Omega 3 group it needs the 'parent' Omega 3 fatty acid, Alpha Linolenic Acid (ALA). In order to make Omega 6 fatty acids it needs the 'parent' Linoleic Acid (LA).

- **Omega 3:** Alpha Linolenic Acid (ALA) is converted by the body into eicosapentaenoic acid (EPA) and decosahexaenoic acid (DHA). Unfortunately this conversion process is not very efficient and some scientists believe that as little as 1% of the Alpha Linolenic Acid we consume ends up as DHA and EPA. This 1% conversion rate decreases even more as we get older. Luckily both DHA and EPA can also be obtained directly from our food so we need to obtain a lot of DHA and EPA as well as ALA from our diet in order to make up for this poor conversion process. Unfortunately the modern Western diet does not provide a very good source of Omega 3 fats.

- **Omega 6:** Linoleic Acid (LA) is converted into Gamma-linolenic acid (GLA) and Arachidonic Acid (AA). Unlike ALA it is readily converted into GLA and AA and our Western diet provides an abundant source of Linoleic Acid.

In the early 1900's most of the fat in our diet was saturated or monounsaturated. It came mainly from butter, lard, beef fat, coconut or palm oil and in some parts of the world olive oil. Over the last three or four decades most of us have been led to believe that saturated fats are bad and that vegetable oils are good. Not true. Any dietary fat or oil can become harmful if it is oxidised and polyunsaturated oils are more likely to be damaged by being oxidised than anything else. Today most of the fat in our diet is polyunsaturated and in the form of soy, corn, sunflower, safflower and canola oil. The detrimental effect these fats have on our health is clear and well established, yet most of us still believe that they are the healthy option.

In all mammals cell tissues are made up mainly of saturated and monounsaturated fats. Omega 3 and Omega 6 fats are only needed in relatively small amounts. What makes polyunsaturated vegetable oils so bad for us is the large amount of them we now consume and as a consequence the residual amount that we have in our bodies.

Saturated Fats:

Under normal conditions the saturated fats found in butter, eggs, cheese and meat are not easily oxidised. The cholesterol and essential fatty acids these foods contain are nutrients that provide the raw materials our bodies need to make a large number of hormones and enzymes as well as vitamin D. They also play a major part in helping to build our body's own antioxidant defence team. Notwithstanding that many of us have been led to believe that cholesterol and saturated fats are 'bad', in reality our bodies are desperately in need of them. They are needed to build brain and nerve tissue, they nourish the immune system, they help regulate our mood and they are one of the building blocks for oestrogen and testosterone.

Contrary to what we have been told, saturated fats are not the "bad guys". They are an essential part of living and when they are replaced by other less healthy fats things can start going wrong. One of the interesting things about them is that to a certain extent our brain in a way 'runs' on them so when they are in short supply it steals them from other parts of our body in order to keep going. Two things that suffer are oestrogen and testosterone, and low levels of these hormones can have an adverse impact on our body and as testosterone levels decline it produces more uric acid.

Monounsaturated Fats:

The monounsaturated fatty acid most commonly found in our food is oleic acid which is the main component of olive oil. It is also found in the oils from almonds, pecans, cashews, peanuts and avocados. Olive oil contains 75% oleic acid, 13% saturated fat in the form of Palmitic acid, 10% omega-6 and 2% omega-3. It is also rich in polyphenols which have antioxidant, anti-inflammatory, anti-clotting and anti-bacterial properties. It is an oil that has withstood the test of time and it is the safest vegetable oil you can use, provided of course that it is consumed in sensible amounts, oils and fats contain a lot of calories.

Polyunsaturated Fats and Oils:

In sharp contrast to saturated and monounsaturated fats, the polyunsaturated fats in vegetable and seed oils are easily oxidised and they undergo further oxidation in a manufacturing process that also damages their molecular structure. This occurs because the seeds and nuts that are used to make the oils are heated to high temperatures, exposed to high pressures and mixed with chemicals and solvents during the manufacturing process. Consumption of such chemically altered oils disrupts our normal metabolism and provides a major source of free radicals. The richer the oil in polyunsaturated fatty acids and the longer it is exposed to heat, light and oxygen, the lower the quality of the oil becomes, the more free radicals in contains and the more damage it is capable of causing.

Because the flavour of poor quality highly oxidised oils can be masked by heavy seasoning, the lowest quality oils are often used in the manufacture of salad dressings and mayonnaise. Ironically, more often than not, these are presented as being the 'healthy' or 'lite' option. Even the premium priced cold-processed oils sold in health food stores can also contain damaging free radicals because as soon as they are extracted and exposed to oxygen and light they begin to oxidise. Contrary to what we are led to believe even "cold pressed" oils are subjected to some heat during the manufacturing process in order to inactivate enzymes that can produce undesirable breakdown products that are toxic to mammals. While they are not heated to the same temperatures as hot pressed oils, a considerable amount of heat is produced by the pressing process itself.

Irrespective of whether they are cold pressed or heat extracted, heating any type of polyunsaturated vegetable oils to high temperatures to fry food will compound the problem. When any oil is heated, the rate of oxidation increases rapidly, doubling with every ten degrees centigrade rise in temperature, so the more the oil is heated the more free radicals are produced. Polyunsaturated oils come complete with their own supply of free radicals plus the free radicals that they have inherited from the manufacturing and cooking process. However, once they are inside our body they undergo a further process of peroxidation and this results in yet more free radicals. The fatty acid or 'lipid' peroxides that result from this have the potential to create an enormous amount of damage when they are incorporated into cell membranes where they wreak havoc, disrupting cell metabolism and ultimately damaging or killing the cell. Our body is traumatised by them and when this happens uric acid is released into the bloodstream and an inflammatory cascade begins. This results in increased oxidative stress and increased pressure on our body's antioxidant defences.

In a typical Western diet around 30% of a days calories come from polyunsaturated vegetable oils. This is an astonishingly high figure and research indicates that this amount is far too high. The best evidence suggests that the daily intake of PUFA's should be around 4% of the total number of calories. No one ever ate oils like this a hundred years ago because they simply did not exist. Where do the oils come from? Salad dressings, mayonnaise, fried foods, chips, fries, cakes, biscuits, processed foods. Its a long list and more often than not we are eating them without even realising it.

Margarine, Shortening and 'Trans Fats'

Is Margarine a healthier option than butter? Well for years we have been told that it is. However, a process called 'hydrogenation' is used to convert polyunsaturated fats that are liquid at room temperature into Trans Fats that are solid at room temperature. In reality Trans Fats are Polyunsaturated Vegetable Oils (PUFA') in their worst possible form and they are found in just about all of the processed food we eat.

The manufacturing process of Hydrogenation is far from being a healthy process and not surprisingly the end result of the process is not a healthy product. Polyunsaturated oils that are already heavy in free radicals from the extraction process are mixed with a catalyst that is then subjected to hydrogen gas in a high pressure, high temperature reactor. Hence 'hydrogenated'. Emulsifiers and starch are then added to improve the consistency and the oil is again subjected to high temperatures in order to steam clean it and remove any unpleasant smells. Bleach, dyes and flavours are then added to make it look like and taste like butter. By the time margarine reaches your table it is a completely unnatural product and hardly the healthy food it is promoted as being! Trans fats are polyunsaturated vegetable oils in their worst possible form.

The high temperatures and chemicals used in the hydrogenation process not only create even more free radicals, they also transform the chemical structure of the oils that are used by changing the position of some of the hydrogen atoms. Hence the name trans fats. As it is almost impossible to remove all of the chemicals used in the manufacturing process, most of these trans fats contain small amounts of toxins as well as a load of free radicals. Because the trans fats mimic naturally occurring fats the body doesn't recognise them as being different and as a consequence they are not excreted. Instead, just like any other naturally occurring polyunsaturated fat they are incorporated into cell membranes where they wreak havoc. The end result is high levels of uric acid and inflammation at the site of the cell death, yet more free radicals and more pressure on our body's antioxidant defences, and this is at a time when the body is being deprived of the raw materials in the form of saturated fats that it needs to make them. A strong correlation between hydrogenated fats and disease was observed as long ago as the 1940's but despite this, more than seventy years on, they are still being promoted as being the 'healthy' option.

Trans Fats in the form of margarine and shortening have the commercially pleasing property of being able to extend a products' shelf life. They are also cheap and because of this they are widely used in manufactured and processed foods. Look on a label and all too often you will see 'hydrogenated vegetable fat' as one of the ingredients. As with the polyunsaturated vegetable oils from which they are derived, no one ever ate food like this years ago because it simply did not exist.

Inflammation and the Inflammatory Cascade

Sounds bad! Well it gets worse. Without getting into the biochemistry in too much detail, there is a complicated interaction between inflammatory messengers, cytokines, prostaglandins and the short lived hormones inside our cells called eicosanoids which can act as either pro-inflammatory and anti-inflammatory compounds. Put simply, the anti-inflammatory eicosanoids draw upon the Omega-3 group of fatty acids in our tissues, EPA and DHA and these put a 'brake' on the inflammation and calm it down. The pro-inflammatory eicosanoids draw on the Omega-6 group of fatty acids GLA and AA and these stimulate the inflammatory response. In order to maintain a proper inflammatory response we need both of these eicosanoids but with high levels of Omega-6 we end up making far too many pro-inflammatory eicosanoids and not enough anti-inflammatory ones.

Omega-3 fats are found abundantly in oily fish, seafood, nuts and a few seeds like flax. To a lesser extent they are also found in meat, dairy products and green vegetables. Omega-6 fats occur naturally in small amounts in nuts and seeds but they are abundant in manufactured vegetable oils and hydrogenated trans fats.

In the good old days when Omega-3 and Omega-6 fats were obtained naturally from food that was unprocessed things were quite well balanced. We were consuming them in a ratio of between one Omega-3 to one Omega-6 or at most one Omega-3 to four Omega-6. With the advent of polyunsaturated vegetable oils this ratio changed dramatically. Because we consume so much vegetable oil and hydrogenated vegetable oil in the form of trans fats, many of us now consume up to twenty or thirty times more Omega-6 than Omega-3 and this can create a highly inflammatory environment within our body. This has major consequences when added to the large amount of other pro-inflammatory foods we are consuming. Polyunsaturated vegetable oils and trans fats are simply fuelling inflammation.

How can we reduce our consumption of PUFA's and Trans Fats?

Switch to butter and olive oil. They are healthy foods that have both stood the test of time. Goose fat and lard are also alternatives but take care and use all of these in moderation. Fat is a high energy food so it contains a lot of calories; just 8 grams of butter contains 50 kcal and 1 tablespoon olive oil contains 120 kcal. If you want to use salad dressings make your own; flax and hemp seed oils are good as well as olive oil. When you buy any oil make sure you read the label carefully and buy only oils that have been 'cold pressed'. They are still damaged but less damaged than the hot pressed oils. Oil that is in a dark bottle is best as it protects the oil from sunlight and also keep the oil in the fridge as this also reduces the rate at which it oxidises.

A note about labelling legislation as this varies enormously between countries. In the EU cold pressed means just that, but in many other countries labels are simply marketing tools that can say more or less anything.

Which foods contain PUFA's and trans fats?

In terms of trans fats we are back to the old chestnut of biscuits, cookies, cakes, more or less anything that is processed, as well as margarines, 'spreadable' butter, non dairy creamers. The number of products containing polyunsaturated vegetable oils is enormous; crisps, chips, fries, salad dressings, mayonnaise, anything that is fried commercially. It really is staggering how these unhealthy oils have stealthily found their way into our food and even more staggering how they are so often presented as 'the healthy' option.

An interesting quotation that is worth keeping in mind:

"Nature doesn't make bad fats, factories do... "

Dr Cate Shanahan

Food That Contains Iron:

How can iron possibly be bad for us?

If you suffer from gout the amount of iron in your blood is probably quite high. If you have been consuming a typical western diet it is unlikely to be low. High levels of iron are bad for several reasons. Iron is needed to make Xanthine Oxidase, the last enzyme your body uses in the process of breaking down and converting purines into uric acid. The more Xanthine Oxidase you have the more uric acid your body is able to make. In addition, iron binds to Vitamin C and destroys its ability to work as an antioxidant. As Vitamin C is something the body tries very hard to hang on to, in order to protect the Vitamin C it produces uric acid as this binds to the iron instead of the Vitamin C. This is something of a vicious circle which means that high levels of iron are implicated in stimulating the production of uric acid and it does it in two ways.

Over the years high levels of stored iron slowly damage the pancreas and this affects its ability to produce insulin. This ultimately leads to insulin resistance and diabetes, both of which are known to raise levels of uric acid by increasing the 're-uptake' of uric acid after it is filtered out. As a consequence this reduces the overall amount of uric acid that is excreted. Also, when the body is in a state of "iron overload" the iron can lead to the production of hydroxyl and peroxyl radicals, some of the most highly reactive and dangerous free radicals that occur in our bodies and these can damage cell membranes and give rise to extreme oxidative stress.

Too Much Iron: 'Iron Overload'

Iron is an essential nutrient and for years a lack of it caused one of the most common nutritional deficiencies, anaemia. However, in the Western world more attention is being paid these days to the opposite problem, iron overload, which has been linked to an increased risk of diabetes, coronary heart disease and cancer. In a recent study of 1,000 white Americans between the age of 67 and 96, 13% had levels of iron that were considered high and only 3% were considered to be deficient in iron. In the western world iron deficiency in men and post menopausal women is rare.

Our body handles iron very carefully, to the extent that it even recycles it from old red blood cells. Recycling is essential as the human diet historically contained only just enough iron to replace the small amount that is lost each day. Our body is also able to regulate the 'uptake' of iron; the less iron you have the more iron your body absorbs, likewise the more iron you have the less it absorbs. Because iron is so important our body guards its store of iron very carefully, so carefully in fact that it has no way of excreting it. Each day we only need a trace amount of iron to replace the tiny amount that we lose. Even for an adult man this is as little as 1mg to 2mg a day. Because the body is unable to completely shut down the absorption process the more iron we consume and absorb from our food the higher the level of stored iron becomes. Short of a blood donation, the body just can't get rid of it.

Even without a rare genetic disorder (Hemochromatosis) that leads to the accumulation of very high levels of iron, stored iron can cause health problems. In a 10 years study of 32,000 women, those who consumed the most iron, and as a consequence had the highest levels of stored iron, were nearly three times more likely to have diabetes than those with the lowest levels of iron. In another study of 38,000 men, those who consumed the most iron had a 63% greater risk of developing diabetes. This begs the question of whether is it the actual iron or other things in the food containing the iron that was causing the diabetes. It could also be that other foods consumed with the iron rich food, a steak with chips or fries for instance, were contributing to the problem. However, other studies have since shown that when people with high levels of stored iron donate blood on a regular basis, their insulin sensitivity and risk of diabetes diminishes. Why? Put simply, iron overload damages the pancreas and affects its ability to produce insulin, so the end result for some is insulin resistance and diabetes, both of which can cause an increase in levels of uric acid.

Where Does The Iron In Our Diet Come From?

Meat, fish, poultry, eggs and vegetables all contain iron. However there are two different types of iron. HEME iron is a type of iron that is derived from red blood cells and it is only found in meat, fish and poultry. Non HEME iron is found in vegetables and fruit as well as animal products. HEME iron is much more easy to absorb than non HEME iron. Whereas between 15% and 30% of HEME iron is absorbed, only about 5% of non HEME iron finds its way into the blood. Interestingly, the uptake of the non HEME iron is much better regulated by the body than the uptake of the HEME iron, so the accumulation of iron and iron 'over load' is more likely if your diet is high in the iron found in animal products.

Various factors can influence the way in which iron is absorbed and not least of these is gender. Pre menopausal women absorb iron much more efficiently than men; from a similar meal they will absorb around three times as much as a man and when they are pregnant this figure can increase to around nine times. Vitamin C, some of the proteins found in meat, and acids naturally present in many fruits and vegetables can all increase the absorption of the non HEME iron found in vegetables, sometimes by as much as 85%. Alcohol and sugar consumption enhance the absorption of both types of iron. While Vitamin C has a neutral effect on how HEME iron is absorbed, some vegetables like spinach, that contain oxalic acid can interfere with and slow down the absorption of HEME iron. High fibre whole grains that contain phytates and foods that are high in calcium also reduce the amount of iron that is absorbed. So it would appear that the more vegetables you eat the less HEME iron your body is able to take on board. Where else does the iron in our diet come from? Probably as a legacy from the past, when dietary iron was in short supply, most manufactured food is now enriched with iron; flour, breakfast cereals, breads, pasta, even infant formula and baby foods are all fortified with iron and many of us also take daily vitamin supplements without realising that they also contain iron.

Not so long ago, before farming became a semi industrialised process with huge animal feeding operations, the price of meat and poultry was high. Only the wealthy could afford to eat it every day. For most people meat was something of a luxury that was only consumed once or twice a week and even then, it was only consumed in modest amounts. However, with the advent of intensive farming methods the price of meat dropped and as a consequence consumption has soared. In 1961 the world's total meat supply was estimated to be 71 million tons. By 2007, it had risen to 284 million tons. When you allow for world population growth and real changes in global GDP, this represents a 70% increase. Per capita consumption has more than doubled over that period. In developing countries it has risen twice as fast, doubling in the last 20 years.

Americans are now consuming close to 276 pounds of meat, poultry and fish per person per year and getting on for half of this is red meat. Australians are consuming almost as much but in Luxembourg the figure is even higher; 300lbs or just over 140kg per person per year. Not surprisingly India has the lowest consumption of meat at 7 pounds, just over 3 kilos a person. 276 pounds of meat a year works out at just under 12 ounces or 350 grams of meat, poultry or fish a day. Red meat contains around 3.7mg iron per 100 grams, fish and poultry around 1.3mg. So if you consume 350 grams of animal protein a day that's just under 13mg from red meat and 4.5mg from poultry and fish. As getting on for half of our animal protein consumption is from red meat, that averages out at around 8.75mg of iron a day.

How much iron do we need on a daily basis?

Well, we know that a healthy man only actually needs between 1mg and 2mg of iron a day, so to allow for the fact that only some of the iron we consume is absorbed the recommended daily guideline is 8mg a day for men and post menopausal women and 18mg a day for pre menopausal women. When you look at these figures 8.75mg a day from animal protein doesn't look too bad. However, other foods like bread, breakfast cereals, flour and pasta are all fortified with iron. Because so many nutrients are taken out in the milling and refining process, in most countries white bread is fortified with enough iron to bring it to within 80% of the amount of iron that is naturally found in whole grain bread, 3.6mg per 100 grams. Now because the fibre and phytates in whole grain bread reduce the absorption of iron, this amount of iron isn't too much of a problem, but in white bread there is very little fibre and no phytates. An average slice of white bread weighs around 70 grams and that means that it contains 2.5mg of iron. How much bread does the average person consume each day? A lot more than one slice. Breakfast cereal contains anything upwards of 10mg of iron per 100 grams. Even with the recommended serving of just 30 grams this means that 3.3mg of iron are added to the daily iron load and many of us actually eat portions of breakfast cereal that are nearer to 50 or 70 grams. If you include bread, pasta and other fortified foods it is easy to see how the recommended daily allowance for iron of 8mg a day is easily exceeded. Just one average portion of animal protein, 2 slices of white bread and 30 grams of breakfast cereal will deliver just over 19mg, more than twice the recommended daily amount. How much of this iron is actually absorbed is another matter, but it is clear that with such an abundant supply of iron slowly, over a number of years, it is easy for iron to accumulate to a level that will ultimately cause health problems.

So with the widespread consumption of large quantities of animal proteins, iron enriched processed foods and a diet that is low in vegetables, fruit and fibre, many people in the Western world now have levels of stored iron that are higher than they should be. In addition to stimulating Xanthine Oxidase and the production of uric acid, this iron also increases the risk of developing insulin resistance and diabetes, both of which reduce the excretion of uric acid and contribute to the development of hyperuricemia and gout.

Sometimes excess iron can behave badly

When we are overloaded with free radicals or when certain essential vitamins and minerals are in short supply, our body does not work quite as well as it should. When our body has too much iron, the iron itself can sometimes cause problems.

Iron is essential for life. It is used in our blood to transport oxygen around our body. It is used in the conversion of sugar, fats and proteins into something called Adenosine Triphosphate (ATP), the store of energy that is inside all of our cells, and it is an essential constituent of the antioxidant Catalase, one of the antioxidants our body makes.

Because iron is so important to us it has a selective advantage when it competes with other trace elements like zinc, copper and manganese for absorption. As a consequence it is easy for us to become saturated with iron at the expense of these other trace elements. The imbalance between the over absorption of iron and the under absorption of copper has a significant impact on the production of uric acid. Iron activates Xanthine Oxidase and stimulates the production of uric acid and copper deactivates it. So as the level of iron increases and the level of copper decreases more uric acid is made.

Some trace elements play an important role in our body's own endogenous antioxidant defences and when this happens iron can cause antioxidants to malfunction by taking the place of the trace elements they need to make them work effectively. One of these is Superoxide Dismutase, an important antioxidant that is involved in the process of mopping up the superoxide free radicals that are produced when uric acid is made. Superoxide Dismutase needs zinc and copper, so when levels of iron are high these trace elements are in short supply and there is not enough active Superoxide Dismutase. The superoxide radicals remain unchecked. Superoxide Dismutase is not the only endogenous antioxidant that high levels of iron can have an adverse effect on. While iron is needed for our bodies to make the antioxidant Catalase, the antioxidants glutathione peroxidase and metallothionein both need copper, so when it is short supply because the body has absorbed iron in preference to copper, their effectiveness is also reduced.

The HEME and non HEME iron that we consume in our food is in the form of ions. These ions are 'positively' charged particles and they need something to attach themselves to in order to 'neutralise' this positive charge. When molecules of various proteins 'bind' to them they are neutralised. The terms 'liganded' or 'chelated' are used to describe this process. Both uric acid and Vitamin C have the ability to chelate and bind to iron as well as other metal ions. Some of the antioxidants we obtain from our food are also known to be able to do this. However, if the inactivation process is for some reason incomplete and the iron ions still retain their charge they can react and produce some of the body's most dangerous free radicals.

This is where things start to get a bit technical. Superoxide and hydrogen peroxide free radicals are generated in the body through various biochemical processes. Under normal conditions these two free radicals rarely interact. However, in the presence of certain metal ions, particularly iron, a sequence of reactions can take place and this produces something called Hydroxyl radicals. Hydrogen peroxide produces the hydroxyl radical by removing an electron from the metal ion, but a sort of chain reaction then follows as the metal ion is regenerated by the Superoxide. It is then able to react with more hydrogen peroxide to produce yet more hydroxyl radicals.

Hydroxyl radicals have a very short life, they are highly reactive and they work at a localised level. This makes them very dangerous compounds that are known to damage DNA, cell membranes and amino acids. They can also react with hydrogen peroxide in another chain reaction that produces yet more free radicals, this time in the form of peroxyl radicals. Unlike Superoxide radicals which can be rendered harmless by Superoxide Dismutase, these hydroxyl and peroxyl radicals can not be eliminated by any of the body's own antioxidant enzymes on their own. They need a hefty team of dietary antioxidants as well as our body's own endogenous antioxidants to work together to make them safe. With the lower levels of our body's own antioxidants that is caused by the iron overload, these free radicals are a major source of cell damage and oxidative stress, both of which lead to cell trauma, increased levels of uric acid and inflammation.

How can we reduce the amount of iron we are consuming?

Short of donating blood your body is unable to remove excess iron so you need to reduce your consumption of the foods that contain large amounts of iron; red meat and to a lesser extent poultry. The largest amounts of HEME iron, the iron that is most easily adsorbed and less well regulated by the body, comes from red meat. So if you really do want to get on the road to recovery you are going to have to stop eating red meat for a while. If you eat more vegetables your body will absorb less iron but you do need to reduce the overall amount of iron you consume. If you feel unable to cut out meat or animal products completely, change from red meat to poultry and fish. They both contain iron but in much smaller amounts and fish, especially oily fish, is high in the Omega-3 essential fatty acids that are actually good for gout. But remember, many manufactured foods are fortified with iron. For example white flour, breakfast cereals, breads, pasta as well as any vitamin supplements you may be taking all contain added iron. Alternative sources of protein? Well dare I suggest beans, pulses and tofu. They are excellent sources of protein and the diet of many people in this world is based on them. Tofu and other soy products like tempeh are particularly rich in micro nutrients and some of these micro nutrients like isoflavones are thought to have powerful anti-inflammatory properties and your body needs anti-inflammatory food.

CARBOHYDRATES

When consumed in excess all types of carbohydrates are bad, irrespective of whether the carbohydrate is the starch found in bread, rice and potatoes or sugar in all its forms and disguises. Incidentally alcohol (ethanol) is metabolised in exactly the same way as the sugar fructose, so when it comes to gout alcohol effectively counts as carbohydrates.

Why are carbohydrates bad for us?

Our ancestors, the early hunter gatherers, are thought to have consumed between 80 and 100 grams of starchy carbohydrates a day and these carbohydrates would have been in a complex unrefined form. It is estimated that the typical Western diet contains between 350-600 grams of carbohydrate a day, a massive increase of between 500% and 750% and our bodies are just not designed to cope with it. If you have gout you will almost certainly also have hyperuricemia as cases of gout without hyperuricemia are rare. It also means that you will either be insulin resistant or near to becoming insulin resistant. This affects your body's ability to excrete uric acid and as a consequence levels of uric acid increase. Insulin resistance also leads to a state of chronic inflammation and an environment in which the oxidation of fats and lipid peroxidation can take place at an alarming rate.

Across the population insulin levels are rising

Our bodies produce insulin when we consume and metabolise carbohydrates. But what exactly are carbohydrates? Most of us immediately think of pasta, rice, bread and potatoes but carbohydrates come in many disguises. They are one of the most abundant biological molecules and they fulfil many roles. The food we eat supplies us with carbohydrates in two different forms, starch and sugar. Both of these contain fibre and cellulose. Starches and sugars provide us with energy. Fibre and cellulose provides us with the 'bulk' our digestive systems need to work efficiently. With the exception of the sugar fructose, all carbohydrates, irrespective of whether they are starch or sugar, are digested and metabolised to into glucose and this is used throughout our body as a source of energy.

The amount of insulin circulating in our bodies is directly related to both the amount of carbohydrates we consume and the 'form' in which they are consumed. When they are complex they take longer to digest and metabolise. The more carbohydrates we consume the more insulin we need to keep glucose levels properly regulated. Over time cells become resistant to insulin so the pancreas needs to produce more in order to keep things in check. In the end it is not able to produce enough insulin to control the amount of glucose in the blood. Eventually Metabolic Syndrome develops and then Type II diabetes. If the pancreas becomes totally exhausted and loses it ability to produce insulin Type I insulin dependent diabetes can result. It is not uncommon for adults to be somewhere between these two extremes, producing more insulin than normal but still able to keep their blood glucose within limits.

High levels of insulin correlate to glucose intolerance, insulin resistance and diabetes. Between one in three and one in four people in the west is now thought to be suffering from one of these conditions. Persistently high levels of insulin also block the breakdown of fat and this leads to weight gain and above normal body weight. This is close to becoming an epidemic even amongst children.

Carbohydrates are natural foods. They become unnatural when they are in a form, concentration or quantity that is not found in nature. In nature sweet and starchy things like fruit and carbohydrates are rare and they are usually only available for a short time of the year. The reason a lot of us crave sugar and carbohydrates is that from an evolutionary perspective they are quite rare nutrients and it was a good idea to eat a lot of them when you could. For early man fruit and tubers containing carbohydrate were usually only around in the autumn so we are wired to eat a lot, store them as fat and use the fat to help us to survive the winter when food was scarce.

Natural unrefined unprocessed carbohydrates come with loads of fibre, vitamins, minerals, water, antioxidants and phytonutrients. The water fills you up and the fibre slows the rate at which the carbohydrates are absorbed in the digestive tract and converted to glucose. This means that they create less of a 'sugar spike' in the blood and this has a direct impact on the amount and rate at which insulin is produced. The vitamins, antioxidants and phytonutrients are valuable as they are essential for our bodies to function properly and they also help prevent and repair cell damage.

Starchy Carbohydrates

In addition to the amount of carbohydrate that we consume, the type of carbohydrate has also changed. Instead of complex 'whole' carbohydrates that contain large amounts of fibre and micro nutrients we are now consuming highly refined carbohydrates and this has as much effect on insulin levels as the amount of carbohydrate itself. The slower the rate at which carbohydrates are absorbed and converted to glucose the less insulin the body needs to produce to regulate blood glucose levels.

Where do these refined carbohydrates come from in our diet? Bread, cakes, biscuits/cookies, breakfast cereals, crisps, chips/fries, rice, pasta; the list is endless and the carbohydrates are invariably 'empty', over refined and very low in nutritional value.

How can we regulate our insulin?

As an initial step, try to reduce your consumption of carbohydrates to between 50 and 100 grams a day. This sounds a bit extreme but it is the first step on the road to recovery. You need to regulate your insulin, get it under control and reset your insulin sensitivity. Once your insulin sensitivity is under control you will be able to relax a bit and increase the amount of carbohydrate you eat to between 100 and 150 grams a day.

This is easier said than done as many foods contain 'hidden' carbohydrates. When we think about carbohydrates we automatically think of bread, rice, pasta, potatoes and cakes. But remember, fruit and vegetables also contain carbohydrates in the form of starch and sugar. Banana is a great food that you should most definitely be eating. Just remember that it is quite high in carbohydrates and these carbohydrates are in the form of sugar. Know how much you are eating, so weigh the banana and other fruit.

Stop eating packaged and processed foods. Most of us eat them every day. They are loaded with over refined carbohydrates and have little to no nutritional value. Switch to complex whole grain carbohydrates and food that is made from them, whether cracked, crushed or rolled. They contain the essential parts and nutrients of the entire grain or seed and these are needed to build your body's antioxidant defence team. Change from white and wholemeal bread to whole grain bread, pumpernickel, rye or spelt. Better still, have a go at making your own bread using spelt and rye flour. It doesn't have to be yeast bread either. Soda bread is great and it only takes minutes to prepare. But take care. A slice of bread contains a lot of carbohydrate, so eat it in moderation.

Use cooking methods that reduce the glycemic index of the carbohydrate foods you eat. Rather than eating carbohydrate vegetables as soon as they are cooked, leave them to cool to room temperature or keep them in the fridge overnight. This changes the structure of the starch they contain and it leaves them with a much lower glycemic index. Lemon juice, lime juice and vinegar all slow down the rate at which carbohydrates are digested, absorbed and converted into glucose.

Tips:

We live in a culture that expects to have a portion of carbohydrates with each meal and moving away from this takes some doing. Try substituting lightly cooked mashed cauliflower for rice. Shredded cabbage 'tagliatelle' works well. Beans like borlotti, fava beans, chickpeas and butter beans are a great source of protein and fibre and they contain far less carbohydrate than the same weight of potatoes, rice or pasta.

SUGAR & HIGH FRUCTOSE CORN SYRUP

Why is sugar and high fructose corn syrup so bad?

Because your body simply does not need sugar, irrespective of what form it comes in. It can make all the glucose it needs from the carbohydrates you consume, even when you have reduced your carbohydrate intake. All consuming sugar and high fructose corn syrup will do is increase your insulin sensitivity, increase the amount of uric acid you are producing and reduce the amount of uric acid you are excreting. It will also contribute to a few extra pounds in body weight.

The Carbohydrate Sugar

Man's love affair with sugar goes back a long way and it plays an insidious role in our health. For some reason we are in a way 'wired' to seek it out. But if sugar is bad for us why do we crave it? The short answer is that like other 'tasty foods' sugar stimulates the same centres in our brain that respond to heroin and cocaine and just like these drugs it has a very pronounced effect. In reality sugar acts on our brain almost like an addictive drug.

Why this happens is interesting as it comes from a time in our evolutionary past when as a result of climate change sugar, in the form of fruit, was only available for a short time of the year. Millions of years ago our early ancestors lived in a tropical climate and were able to eat fruit containing sugar throughout the year. As they moved into Eurasia and the climate cooled the forests became deciduous and fruit was only available for a short time of the year. This resulted in hungry near starving apes and a species that was in decline. At some point a mutation occurred and this made some of the apes extremely efficient at processing the fructose that was found in the seasonal fruit. Even small amounts could be metabolised and very quickly stored as fat. This gave these apes a huge survival advantage. They ate a lot of fruit while they could, put on fat and used the fat to help them survive when food was scarce.

Today all apes, including humans, have this mutation. Our bodies have evolved to survive on very little sugar. So when sugar, especially in its refined form, is available we get fat because we are in some way 'wired' to seek it out and we eat far too much of it.

A Brief History of Sugar.

In reality sugar is one of the first 'manufactured' foods. It was first domesticated on the island of New Guinea about 10,000 years ago. The raw sugar cane was chewed and it is thought that the juice extracted from the cane was used in religious ceremonies. Sugar spread slowly from island to island reaching mainland Asia around 1,000BC. By 500AD it had reached India where it was used as a medicine. By 600AD it had spread to Persia and when the Arab armies conquered Persia they took a love of sugar and the knowledge of how to make it back to the Middle East. As the Arab Empire grew, wherever they went sugar went with them and they more or less turned sugar refining into an industry.

Probably the first Europeans to come across sugar were the Crusaders and the first sugar began reaching Europe in small amounts. It was regarded as a spice. It was expensive and only consumed by the wealthy. Some enterprising Crusaders saw an opportunity and began farming and processing sugar cane in small quantities in Cyprus but as the Crusades ended the supplies from the Arabs diminished new sources of supply were needed. The hunt was on to find places where sugar cane could be grown and it soon found its way via the Canary and Cape Verde Islands to the Caribbean. As more sugar cane was planted and refined the price of sugar fell and as the price fell so consumption and demand increased. The rest, as they say, is history.

In 1700 the average Englishman consumed 4 pounds of sugar a year. By 1800 he was eating 18 pounds a year and by 1870 consumption had risen to 47 pounds. By 1900 we were consuming 100 pounds a year. Today, about 25 percent of people on a typical 'Western Diet' consume around 95 kilograms or getting on for 200 pounds of sugar a year and for most of us this is more than our body weight. Sounds impossible? Well not when you consider that a 12 ounce can of 'regular' soft drink can contain up to 10 teaspoons of sugar, a massive 40 grams which is just under one and a half ounces.

So what exactly is sugar?

First and foremost sugar is a natural food. It only becomes unnatural when it is in a form, concentration or quality that is not found in nature. Sugar comes in several forms and many disguises. The most common form is sucrose or what we know as table sugar. This is a 'dissacharide', a compound that is made up of one molecule of glucose that is linked to one molecule of fructose. So it contains 50% glucose and 50% fructose. When it is metabolised it is converted into separate molecules of glucose and fructose. These are both simple sugars or 'monosaccharides'. There is a third monosaccharide galactose. All other types of sugar are made from these three monosaccharides.

A voice in the wilderness

In the 1960's a British nutrition expert called John Yudkin conducted a series of experiments on animals and people that showed that high amounts of sugar in their diet led to high levels of fat and insulin in the blood, risk factors he believed to be for heart disease and diabetes. But Yudkin's message was drowned out by the chorus of other scientists who were blaming the rising rates of obesity, heart disease and diabetes on the high levels of cholesterol that resulted from the consumption of too much saturated fat. As a consequence we were told to reduce the amount of saturated fat we were eating and as a result, saturated fat now makes up a smaller proportion of the average American diet than it did 40 years ago. So what filled the gap in fat consumption? Unsaturated fats in the form of vegetable oils and margarine, but despite this the number of people who are overweight or obese has not reduced. In reality it has grown larger and the incidence of heart disease and diabetes has increased at an alarming rate.

Where does sugar come from in our diet?

Sugary soft drinks, biscuits, cakes, cookies, confectionery and surprisingly processed and manufactured foods. Why processed and manufactured foods? Sugar is a wonderful preservative so it is used in large quantities as a preservative. It is also used as a 'browning' agent, on the basis that colour equals flavour. In the west we have become addicted to 'brown', 'caramelised' food.

Fructose and High Fructose Corn Syrup

Fructose, also called fruit sugar, occurs naturally both on its own as a monosaccharide and also as one of the molecules that table sugar, (sucrose), is made from. High Fructose Corn Syrup (HFCS) is a manufactured product that is 55% fructose and 45% glucose. Fructose is the only carbohydrate known to directly increase levels of uric acid and because of this, for many who write about diet and gout, it has become something of a "bête noire", especially when it is in the form of High Fructose Corn Syrup.

Fructose is a simple sugar that is found in varying amounts in fruit and vegetables, either on its own as a monosaccharide or combined with glucose as a disaccharide. When vegetables and fruit are eaten as a 'whole food' and in normal amounts the nutrients, antioxidants, fibre and other compounds that they contain counter any detrimental effect of the fructose as the fibre means that it is absorbed slowly into our bodies. So a small amount of fructose is not a bad thing. In fact, there is some evidence that a little bit may help your body process glucose properly. However, consuming too much fructose, especially when it is in a pure refined form appears to overwhelm the body's ability to process it.

The fructose in HFCS is no different to the fructose found in other foods. Once inside your body fructose works in the same way irrespective of whether it comes from corn syrup, cane sugar, strawberries, onions, or tomatoes. Only the amounts of fructose are different. For example, a cup of chopped tomatoes has 2.5 grams of fructose, a medium size desert apple about 4.5 grams, a 300ml can of non-diet soft drink contains around 23 grams, and a 'super-size' soft drink has about 62 grams. From a health perspective it is strongly recommended that your daily consumption of fructose is less than 25 grams, in other words the amount found in five desert apples or one 300ml can of non diet or 'regular' soft drink. The diets of our ancestors contained only very small amounts of fructose and it was only consumed for short periods of the year when fruit and berries were ripe. They used it to build up their fat reserves for the winter. Today it is estimated that about 10% of the calories in a modern 'Western' diet comes from fructose. Of the 152 pounds of 'sugar' the average American consumes each year 64 pounds is thought to be fructose in the form of High Fructose Corn Syrup.

When it comes to fructose and sugar we are being well and truly 'conned' into thinking that certain foods are healthy when they are not. Honey is presented as a healthy option, presumably because it is 'natural' and contains some beneficial nutrients, but it has about the same fructose to glucose ratio as high fructose corn syrup. Look at the ingredients on the labels of packaged foods and you will invariably see sugar in one form or another. In reality finding manufactured food that does not contain sugar is actually quite difficult. As food manufacturers use the generic term sugar most people have no idea which products fructose is in or how much of it they are consuming.

Why our consumption of fructose has increased at such an alarming rate over the last thirty to forty years is the subject of a considerable amount of speculation. It is easy to become a little cynical about it. In America, because of corn subsidies, High Fructose Corn Syrup became incredibly cheap, much cheaper than conventional sugar. As it is fairly concentrated and in a liquid form that is easy to transport, it quickly found its way into a vast number of the foods we eat every day. Its introduction into the Western diet in 1975 was a multi-billion dollar boon for the corn industry. Almost all manufactured and packaged, processed foods now have sugar added in some form or other and this almost always includes fructose. Just to get some idea of the scale, 240,000 tonnes of fructose are produced each year. A massive amount. Not only is it added to food and drinks, it is also used in large quantities as a 'browning' agent in many manufactured and processed foods and this, in particular, is of great concern as people are unaware that they are consuming sugar. Another issue that needs to be kept in mind is that High Fructose Corn Syrup is almost invariably made from genetically modified corn. Some people have expressed concerns about genetically modified or "GM" foods. While the jury is still out on GM foods it could mean that HFCS brings with it another new set of as yet unknown dangers.

Over the past few years HFCS has been gathering something of a 'bad press' and as a consequence the consumption of both HFCS and sugar is falling slowly. So where do we go from here? Well the corn industry has come up with another product, "crystalline fructose" that is being used in soft drinks. This is produced by allowing fructose to crystallize out from a fructose-enriched corn syrup. This produces a product that is 99.5 percent pure fructose. In other words it contains nearly twice as much fructose as the HFCS currently being used. To make matters worse it is being promoted as being in some way 'healthier', a "pure fruit sugar" that is and better for you than HFCS. Clearly, all the health problems associated with HFCS could become even more pronounced when this product becomes widely used.

There is no doubt that in the Western World we are consuming vast amounts of fructose. Where does fructose come from in our diet? As with all sugars it is present in very large amounts in manufactured foods. In fact it is in almost all of the food that we consume that is not in a 'natural' form. And it shows up is some surprising places, even things that are not 'sweet' like sliced bread and processed meats contain it. Next time you buy a tin of chopped tomatoes check the label. You may be surprised!

How can we reduce the amount of sugar we consume?

Its easier said than done especially if you eat a lot of convenience foods and you drink a lot of non diet carbonated soft drinks. You can cut sugar out of drinks like tea and coffee by using an artificial sweetener. Stevia is the current favourite, but better still, try to retrain your palette. It is not easy but there are some very helpful web sites that can help.

The difficult part about cutting out sugar and High Fructose Corn Syrup is that so many foods contain them; ice cream, mayonnaise and salad dressings are loaded with them as well as trans fats and even 'ready meals' and TV diners have them added as browning agents. In fact they are used in just about all processed foods as a preservative and 'regular' non diet soft drinks and squashes contain an enormous amount, up to 10 teaspoons of sugar (40 grams !) in a 12 oz or 350cc drink.

There is no easy solution to cutting out sugar and HFCS. You are either going to have to stop consuming these types of food completely or start making your own, without sugar.

Tips:

- Avoid fast foods.
- Substitute fizzy water for carbonated soft drinks. Ignore the stuff on the internet that says carbonated fizzy water is bad for you. It is yet more misinformation. Ten teaspoons of sugar in each can of soft drink damages your health far more than carbonated water.
- Make your own lemonade. If you suffer from gout you need the Vitamin C. Lemonade freezes really well and the Vitamin C is not damaged by freezing. If you need to sweeten it use Stevia instead of sugar.
- Read the labels on food very carefully and beware of the word 'natural'. Remember fructose is a natural sugar!
- Be wary of anything in a box or packet with a long shelf life. Sugar and fructose is often used as a preservative.

FRUIT JUICE & SMOOTHIES

The commercial ones that you buy in the Supermarket.

Why are fruit juice and smoothies bad for us?

Because they contain enormous amounts of both fructose and glucose as well as preservatives. They also often contain flavouring and colouring agents. They are not a healthy way to start your day and they are most certainly not one of your "5 a day".

Fruit juice is widely promoted as being one of your “5 a day” and a healthy way to start your day. Not true. Notwithstanding that the processing of these juices strips away most of their nutritional value, they contain a lot of fructose and no fibre. A 100 gram portion of a whole orange contains 1.5grams of fibre and 6.4 grams of sugar, of this sugar 1.9 grams is in the form of fructose. A 100 gram portion of orange juice however contains no fibre and 10 grams sugar, of this sugar 3 grams is in the form of fructose. Doesn't sound too bad? Well it does when you consider that the average orange weighs about 150 grams and the average glass of fruit juice is 300ml or 300 grams. The whole orange provides 2.2 grams of fibre and 9.6 grams of sugar of which 1.9 grams is fructose while the orange juice provides no fibre and 30 grams of sugar and 9 grams of this is fructose. In other words 3 times as much sugar and around 4 times as much fructose. If you are aiming to reduce your daily intake of carbohydrates to between 50 and 100 grams just one glass of fruit juice will account for a very large proportion of it.

How?

Eat whole fruit instead of fruit juice; apples, oranges, cranberries, anything the fruit juice is made from. You will be getting the full benefit of the fruit as well as the fibre and a load of antioxidants. There is an old saying that if you are not hungry enough to eat an apple then you are not hungry. You will get far more satisfaction from the 'crunch factor' of one apple than drinking a glass of apple juice that contains the fructose equivalent of three or four apples.

In terms of smoothies, make your own using fruit and natural unsweetened low fat yoghurt, which incidentally is a very good 'gout friendly' food. Low fat dairy products actually help you excrete uric acid. Use the whole fruit whenever possible. If necessary, buy a small blender. Smoothies freeze really well and as the antioxidants in the fruit is not damaged by freezing make them in large quantities. Just take them out of the freezer and leave them to thaw out overnight in the fridge.

FRYING, GRILLING & ROASTING FOOD

Cooking Food at High Temperatures.

One of the most intriguing aspects of the modern 'Western' diet is the high heat at which so much of our food is cooked. We appear to be addicted to browned, crisp and caramelised food. We fry food in fat or oil, we grill it, we BBQ it and we roast and bake it in hot ovens. The effect that these cooking methods have on our food is immense. None of the food we eat, irrespective of whether it is of animal or plant origin, is designed to withstand cooking at such high temperatures and as a consequence its nutritional content and chemical structure both suffer.

Why do we cook food? Well, while some food can be eaten in its raw, natural state, sometimes cooking is needed in order to:

- increase the amount of nutrients or energy we are able to absorb from the food
- make the food easier to digest
- make food safe to eat by killing bacteria
- tenderise foods that would otherwise be tough and unpleasant to eat
- increase the length of time the food can be kept for

Cooking also has the benefit of sometime improving the taste and flavour of food and making it look more appetising.

What are the consequences of cooking at high temperatures?

Nutritional research is only just starting to catch up with the consequences of our high temperature cooking methods and our addiction to 'browned', 'caramelised' and 'crisp' foods. We know that when oils are heated they oxidise and produce free radicals; the higher the temperature the greater the number of free radicals.

But this isn't the only thing that happens. Cooking at high temperatures, even in the absence of oil, can transform otherwise healthy foods into unhealthy compounds that can cause serious damage to our cells and the DNA within the cells. Heterocyclic amines (HCA's), and polycyclic aromatic hydrocarbons (PAH's), Acrylamide and Advanced Glycation End Products (AGE's) that are also called Glycotoxins, are just some of these compounds. When it comes to hyperuricemia and gout the compounds that are of most interest are the Advanced Glycation End products as these affect just about every type of cell in the body. They are also thought to be a major factor in some age related diseases and they are known to be linked to insulin resistance, diabetes and impaired kidney function, all of which have an impact on both the generation of uric acid and the way our body is able to excrete it.

What are AGE's and where do they come from?

Advanced Glycation End products come from two sources, our bodies and our food. Our bodies produce them as part of normal metabolism. Carbohydrates, irrespective of whether they are simple or complex, are metabolised into glucose and used by our body as a source of energy. However, a small amount of this glucose is glycated to form AGE's. As we get older AGE's are produced in greater numbers and they are also produced in greater numbers if we have higher than normal amounts of glucose in our blood. Scientists studying diabetes have known about the existence of AGE's for years. They have also known that sugars like fructose are glycated ten times faster than glucose. With the dramatic increase in the consumption of sugar, the number of people with high levels of blood sugar and as a consequence high levels of AGE's has increased dramatically over recent years.

Dietary AGE's form as food browns during cooking, primarily when foods high in protein or fat are subjected to high temperatures. When you fry a piece of steak or cook it under the grill you are creating a chemical reaction called a Maillard reaction. This occurs when some of the sugars, fats and proteins in the food react together when they are exposed to high temperatures. The end result are glycotoxins or AGE's. While cooking in dry heat produces the most AGE's, pasteurisation, smoking and microwaving all produce them. Because the beans from which they are made are roasted even coffee and chocolate contain them. The higher the roasting temperature and the longer the roasting time the more AGE's they contain. Any food that contains sugars, fats and proteins is fair game. One of the worrying things about AGE's is that for most of us the browning effect they come from enhances the flavour of food. As a consequence they increase our appetite and this encourages us to eat more. It is not surprising that the food manufacturing industry has taken this interesting characteristic on board and now adds sugar in various forms to certain foods in order to enhance their colour and flavour and entice us to eat more; biscuits, baked goods, ready meals and colas all contain them.

Why should we worry about AGE's?

Once inside the body AGE's can damage cells, tissues and organs and the trauma this damage causes increases levels of uric acid and inflammation. They can also accelerate the general ageing process. The sulphated mucopolysaccharides that form part of the connective tissue that lubricates our joints are known to reduce and breakdown as we get older leaving residual calcium ions that have the potential to seed monosodium urate crystals. The total state of oxidative stress and age related damage is proportional to the dietary intake of AGE's and the consumption of sugar, in all its disguises. One other thing that we should really worry about is that high levels of AGE's are linked to decreased levels of testosterone, even in non diabetic men, and decreased levels of testosterone are linked to increased levels of uric acid and gout.

It is estimated that the standard American diet now contains about 10,000 and 16,000 kU of AGEs each day. This is three times higher than the safety limit advised by professional organisations. Most scientists agree that about ten per cent of the AGE's in our food are absorbed and of this 10%, it takes about three days for the body to excrete around a third of them. The remaining two thirds are not excreted. This means that as they slowly accumulate, there are plenty left hanging around in the body to cause trouble.

What can we do about them?

Different foods produce different amounts of AGE's and different cooking methods also create different amounts. For example, if you fry, grill or roast a 90gram chicken breast it will generate between 4,000 to 9,000 units of AGE's. If you steam, boil or stew it it will produce about 1,000. As a general rule, because they contain less protein, vegetables produce fewer AGE's than animal based products. The more raw foods we eat the lower the number of AGE's. Interestingly, lemon juice and vinegar used as marinades decease the formation of AGE's. So by changing cooking methods, marinading your meat and fish in lemon juice or vinegar and eating less animal protein we can reduce the amount of AGE's we are exposing our bodies to.

There is no doubt that cooking methods produce damaging substances. While they are not themselves free radicals, AGE's damage cells and this damage increases levels of uric acid, gives rise to inflammation and this in turn increases the load of free radicals the body has to cope with. High levels of AGE's are known to be linked to oxidative stress, insulin resistance, diabetes and reduced levels of testosterone and all of these are not a good idea if you suffer from gout.

How can we reduce the number of AGE's we consume?

Different foods produce different amounts of AGE's and different cooking methods also give rise to different amounts. Frying, grilling and roasting create the most, whereas boiling, steaming and braising the least. High protein meats, poultry and fish create more than vegetables although chips and fries also contain them.

The more raw foods we eat the less AGE's we consume and by marinading food in lemon juice or vinegar you can reduce the number of AGE's that form. Changing our cooking methods and eating less animal protein will reduce the amount of AGE's our bodies are exposed to. But be aware that manufactured foods all contain them, even seemingly innocuous things like flaked breakfast cereals, soy sauce, flavourings and dressings.

ALCOHOL

Beer, Lager, Cider, Wine & Spirits

When it comes to gout the consumption of alcohol is and always will be a hot topic. Man has consumed alcohol in various forms for thousands of years. Even primitive man unknowingly consumed it when he ate fruit that was partially fermented. Our bodies also make small amounts of alcohol as part of normal daily living. However, once man became urbanised and was unable to safely drink water from streams and wells the brewing of beer made water safe. While wine was the drink of the rich and privileged, beer was the every day drink for all classes of people. Men, women and even children consumed beer and it was often consumed in quantities that to us are astounding. There is plenty of documentary evidence to support this. Notwithstanding that modern beer, at between 3% and 5%, is much stronger than the 1% to 2% 'small beer' that was consumed then, when drunk in large quantities it still amounts to a lot of alcohol. Records show that in Coventry in the 16th Century in England, the average person consumed about 17 pints of ale a week, six times more than the average consumption today. The household records of a 17th Century English stately home show that a groom, who incidentally rose at 5am and went to bed at 9pm, was given;

> *".... beer and bread for his breakfast at 8am, bread, cheese and beer for his lunch at mid day and bacon, beans and beer for his supper at 7pm ....."*

While these household records do not state how much beer was given with each meal the records of the British armed services do. In addition to their rum and lime juice ration, British sailors received a ration of a gallon, 8 pints, of beer a day. Soldiers each received two thirds of a gallon. As a sailor's beer was usually brewed on board ship we know little about its alcohol content. We do however know about a soldiers' beer. This was in fact a 'porter' and at 6% this was definitely not a 'small beer'.

It is clear that in the past beer was consumed in quantities that are far in excess of today's guidelines. Yes, the life expectancy of the ordinary man then was much shorter, yet people then were far healthier than they are now. Gout was the disease of the wealthy, not the ordinary man. Almost all epidemiological studies find an association between alcohol, gout and healthy 'non drinking' control groups, but some scientists think that the link is not proven. The exact incidence of alcohol induced gout and hyperuricemia still remains unknown. What is known however is that beer drinkers are more likely to have gout than people who drink spirits and people who drink moderate amounts of red wine interestingly appear to have no increased risk of gout at all.

There is no doubt that there is some form of link between alcohol consumption and gout but what is the link? Well one of the interesting things about alcohol is the way in which it is consumed; different types of alcohol are consumed by different groups of people in different ways. Wine tends to be consumed with a meal that is in dietary terms relatively healthy, whereas beer tends to be consumed either on its own or accompanied by snacks that are often far from healthy. As a population, wine drinkers could simply be healthier, eat better quality foods or simply overall consume less alcohol.

Alcohol can induce hyperuricemia and gout in a number of different ways:-

- All alcoholic drinks, irrespective of whether they are beer, lager, wine or spirits contain ethanol and ethanol is metabolised by the liver in exactly the same way as fructose. So when you consume alcohol you are effectively consuming fat. In addition, most alcoholic drinks also contain sugar in some shape or form, so as well as increasing the carbohydrate load and insulin production, the sugar provides unwanted calories that can ultimately end up as fat. As an example, beer contains a sugar called maltose. In a pint of beer there are about 30 grams of maltose and this means a pint of beer contains around 350 kcals. Red wine however contains very little sugar so one 125ml glass of red wine contains only around 100 calories.

- Irrespective of whether it is in the form of beer, lager, wine or spirits, alcohol is a diuretic and diuretics increase the amount of water we excrete. As a consequence when alcohol is consumed in quantity it can lead to dehydration and dehydration can potentially trigger an attack of gout.
- When consumed in large amounts over a short space of time lactic acid is produced as the alcohol is metabolised. The lactic acid can reduce the amount of uric acid excreted by the kidneys.
- Alcohol increases the absorption of iron and as we know, iron stimulates Xanthine Oxidase and the production of uric acid. High levels of iron are also linked to insulin resistance and diabetes, both of which reduce the amount of uric acid excreted.
- Alcohol induces increased levels of iron ions that are not bound to proteins and, as described previously, this can contribute to the formation of dangerous hydroxyl radicals.

As well as promoting the generation of free radicals alcohol also interferes with the body's normal antioxidant defence mechanisms by stripping the body of some of its Vitamin C as well as some of the essential nutrients it needs to make its own endogenous antioxidants. Zinc is of particular interest here as alcohol not only increases the amount of zinc that is excreted, it also reduces the amount of zinc that is absorbed from food. So consuming alcohol on a regular basis, especially if it is consumed in relatively large amounts, can over time lead to low levels of zinc or in extreme cases zinc deficiency. One of our body's endogenous antioxidants that plays a key role in mopping up the superoxide free radicals that are generated when purines are metabolised into uric acid. is Superoxide Dismutase. As this is a zinc based antioxidant low levels of zinc could reduce the amount of Superoxide Dismutase the body is able to make and hence directly lead to increased oxidative stress. The bottom line is that alcohol scores twice. First by increasing the free radical load your body is subjected to and then by reducing your body's ability to cope with the increased load.

As with antioxidants and free radicals, all sources of alcohol are not created equal. Red wine appears to have very little effect on hyperuricemia. Because of the tannins and polyphenols that it contains, red wine actually slows down the absorption of non HEME iron, even though it actually contains moderate amounts of this type of iron. When consumed as part of a meal it slows down the digestion of the meal and this results in more stable blood glucose levels. Because of this, red wine is the key element in what is often described as the 'French Paradox'; the consumption of a rich and potentially unhealthy diet that appears to be made healthy by the inclusion of moderate amounts of red wine. How can red wine make an unhealthy diet healthy? It contains a lot of antioxidants, polyphenols, Resveratrol and quercetin are just some of the them and in some way they appear to balance things out.

So where does this fit into the stereotypical historical view of the gout sufferer? They were the only people who could afford to drink wine and this should in theory have been of benefit to them. We can only assume that the way the wine was made and stored and the vessels from which it was consumed must have played their part.

The consumption of beer has for years been a complete 'no - no' when it comes to gout. But no one is able to provide a convincing reason why it is so much worse than wine or all of the other different types of alcohol. Even when a 'low purine diet' is discounted as an effective way of managing gout, the reason why beer is 'bad' is that it contains the purine Guanosine and Guanosine is one of the purines from which uric acid is made. Confusing!

Well, I have another theory about why beer is bad for gout and I think it is quite convincing. Firstly, like red wine beer contains iron. Around 1.2mg in a pint and that is quite a lot. However, unlike red wine it does not contain anything that inhibits the absorption of the iron so the iron in the beer simply adds to the daily iron load.

Secondly, beer contains lactic acid because lactic acid is produced when beer is brewed. Lactic acid is also produced when alcohol is metabolised, so beer is scoring twice. Lactic acid reduces the amount of uric acid the kidney's excrete, but it also creates a sudden short term acidic 'spike' in the the blood and this can increase the number of calcium ions present and can potentially seed the formation of uric acid crystals.

Last but not least, beer is made from malted barley and barley contains both sugar and protein. When barley is malted it is exposed to high temperatures. As with any type of heat process this produces AGE's, in this case the AGE's are in the form of melanoidins. These melanoidins give the beer its characteristic colour and flavour. The longer the malting process and the higher the temperature, the darker the beer and the higher its AGE content. If the malting process wasn't enough, beer is boiled when it is 'mashed', often for quite a long time and this creates yet more AGE's. The AGE's in beer have exactly the same damaging effect as any other AGEs, leading over time to cell damage, inflammation, insulin resistance, reduced levels of testosterone and ultimately increased levels of uric acid.

When you look at the evidence, alcohol is not a sensible choice if you suffer from hyperuricemia or gout. Apart from contributing to hyperuricemia and potentially triggering a gout flare, it also contains a lot of calories and carrying extra weight will serve only to make a bad situation worse. Just as important though is the simple fact that alcohol weakens your will power, so once you have had one drink it is easy to have another. Then before you know it a little demon takes over and you start 'snacking' as well, usually on the type of junk food that causes gout.

So if you suffer from gout the best advice is to stop drinking completely for at least three months. If you regularly drink beer or lager this is going to be very difficult. Alcohol is not an easy habit to break. In adopting this new eating and lifestyle plan you are going to make a lot of changes and some of these will to you be 'sacrifices'. Just keep saying to yourself that each day without a beer brings you one day nearer to leading a gout free life, and that gout free life could well mean a beer when ever you want one.

If you do not want to stop drinking or you feel unable to, make sure that you drink plenty of water, preferably filtered water, and keep yourself well hydrated. If you do stop drinking, once you have been gout free for several months, then maybe you can experiment and find out if you can tolerate a glass of red wine or a small beer. However, there is no 'one size fits all solution' so the management of alcohol consumption will always remain a personal matter.

FOOD ALLERGIES

Food allergies and "food intolerances"

Gout is a form of inflammatory arthritis so if you suffer from gout your body is in a state of inflammation. One of your key objectives is to reduce that inflammation. Without wishing to sound cranky, one of the reasons you have gout could be that you are 'intolerant' of some of the foods you consume on a regular basis and as a consequence they are contributing to a state of systemic inflammation; wheat gluten, eggs, soy, dairy and some types of nuts, especially peanuts, are known allergens. Lactose intolerance in particular is far more common than we realise. Figures vary but between 5% and 20% of people of Caucasian descent have a level of lactose intolerance and around 35% of the South Sea Islanders have the problem. In people of African decent the figure rises to between 65% and 75%, while in some Asian populations the figures is as high as 90%.

If you suspect that you are sensitive to a specific food or group of foods try eliminating it for at least two weeks. Listen to your body and see if symptoms like lethargy, headaches, flatulence or bloating subside. Tedious and time consuming it may be but its worth it in the long term.

Does History Support This?

Does history support the concept that this food can cause gout?

Notwithstanding that polyunsaturated vegetable oils and trans fats have only recently appeared on the scene, believe it or not it does. Historically gout was the 'disease of kings', a disease that only afflicted the rich, the privileged and the 'men of the cloth'.

Only the rich could afford to eat flour that was in any way refined and 'white'. As you went down through the social scale less wheat and more rye and oatmeal was consumed and the coarser and less refined this 'flour' became. By the time you got to the peasants, the really poor, they couldn't afford flour at all. They ate a sort of meal made from ground up beans or pulses.

The rich ate meat and they ate it in large amounts. The less money you had the less meat and animal protein you consumed. When you got to the poor they ate hardly any. They lived almost exclusively on vegetables. Any animals they had were far too valuable in providing milk or eggs for them to be eaten.

Only the rich roasted their food. They roasted it on spits at a high temperature in front of an open fire. The poor boiled or stewed their food. They used a single large cast iron pot that was hung over the fire. Ovens and cooking ranges only became widely available to the middle and upper classes in early Victorian times. The poor continued to use the 'stew pot' until well into the 19th Century.

Historically carbohydrates generally were in short supply. There were no potatoes, there was no rice and there was certainly no pasta. The carbohydrates that were available were all complex and unrefined. Sugar was an extremely expensive luxury, as was honey. Only the very rich could afford to buy it. With the exception of small amounts of fruit that could be dried or stored, fruit was seasonal. Only the rich could afford the sugar or honey needed to preserve it.

While it is no longer recognised as being one of the causes of gout today, high levels of lead are known to significantly impair kidney function and the amount of uric acid that is excreted. In the homes of the rich and wealthy as well as in the monasteries, pewter was used for tableware and cooking utensils. Lead could easily have leached from the pewter into their food, slowly accumulated in their systems and impaired the way their kidneys worked.

Alcohol. Well this is a paradox. Beer or ale was consumed by all, the poorer classes consuming the most, and it was consumed in amounts that to us are astoundingly high. Spirits as such were extremely rare. Paradoxically it was the rich who drank wine and they were the people suffering from gout, but in those days wine was made in lead lined containers and often preserved and sweetened with lead acetate. Could the mead the monks are reputed to have brewed from honey have anything to do with their gout? It would have contained large amounts of residual sugar as well as lead that was leached from the pots in which it was made.

Summary

"You are what you eat" is an interesting adage that has been around for some time. When it comes to gout you really are what you eat. The evidence is overwhelming. Polyunsaturated vegetable oils, trans fats, too much iron, over refined carbohydrates, and this includes sugar in all its disguises, alcohol and changed cooking methods are all taking their toll. Combined with lifestyle they are major factors in the dramatic increase in not only gout but also many of the other chronic diseases that are becoming so prevalent in the Western World. This means that changes to our diet and the way in which we cook the food we eat can have a positive impact on our health.

Avoid:

- Packaged foods, especially those with a long list of ingredients.
- Food that is fried, BBQ'd, roasted and highly processed. When preparing food select raw, fresh, steamed or boiled foods.

Eliminate:

- Refined polyunsaturated vegetable oils. Any potential health giving properties have been removed during processing and they are overloaded with free radicals and the Omega 6 fats that fuel inflammation.
- Trans Fats and hydrogenated fats. Our bodies have no means of using them and they are a major source of free radicals and inflammation. Together with polyunsaturated vegetable oils they are the single most damaging food in our modern Western Diet.

- Meat and foods like white flour and breakfast cereals that are enriched with iron. Red meat in particular needs to be eliminated, a least in the short term, but if you do eat it try to buy organically reared grass fed meat as this contains more Omega-3 fats than grain fed meat..
- High glycemic index refined carbohydrates; bread, pastries, cakes, biscuits, fruit juice are all rapidly digested and lead to rapid rises in blood glucose levels that create insulin spikes.
- Alcohol. The decision is yours.

Like many things in life food can be addictive and manufactured and processed foods really are addictive, the food manufacturers have made sure of that. Dietary habits are just that, habits, and like all habits they can be changed. We have looked at the food that can cause gout and it is food that many of us we eat on a regular basis. There is no doubt that breaking the eating habits of a lifetime will not be an easy task, but by following these recommendations you will gradually restore your body's natural balance and put yourself on the road to recovery and being able to live a gout free life.

Just remember that the occasional mishap will not spell doom. It is what you do most of the time, not what you do some of the time that matters.

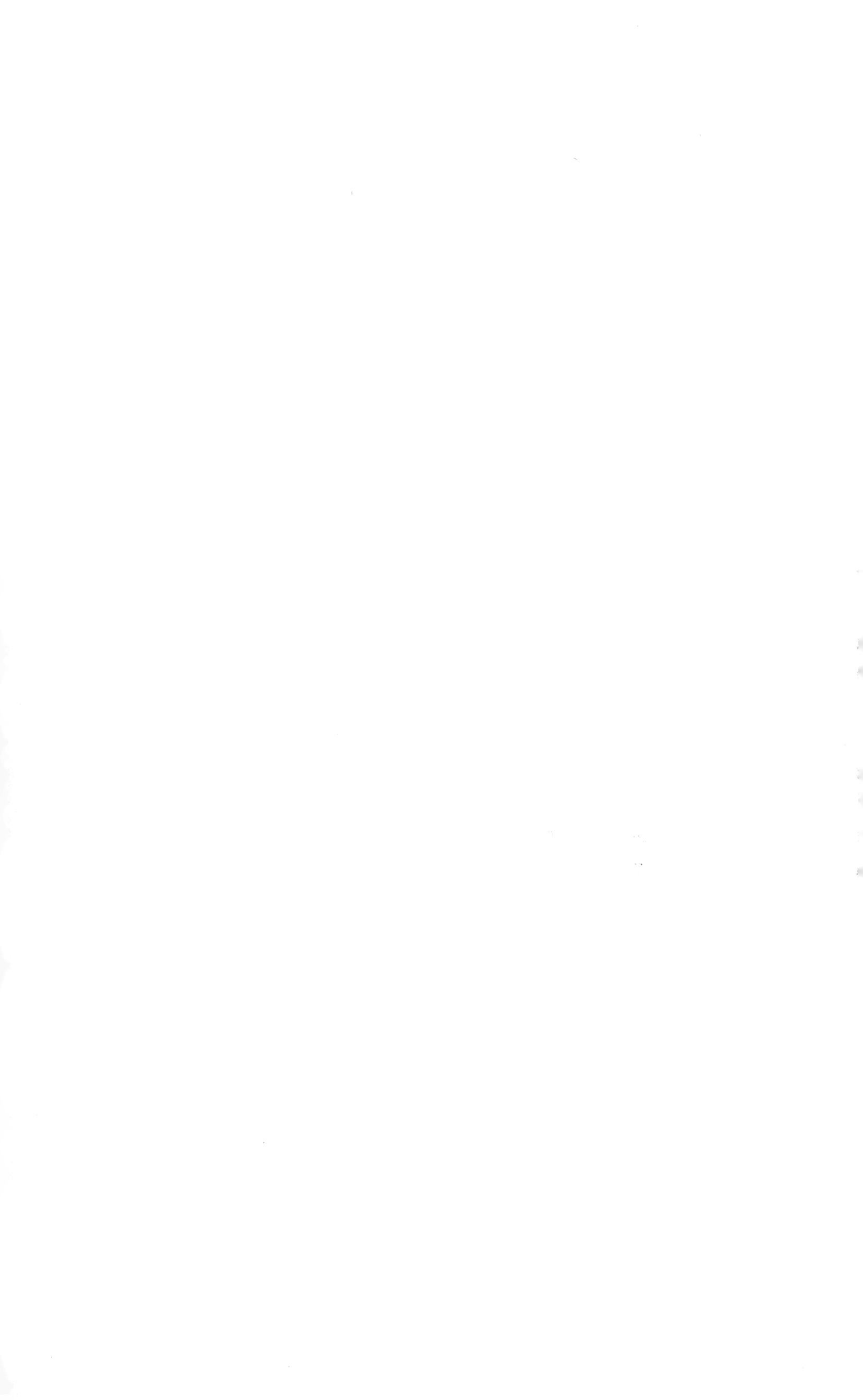

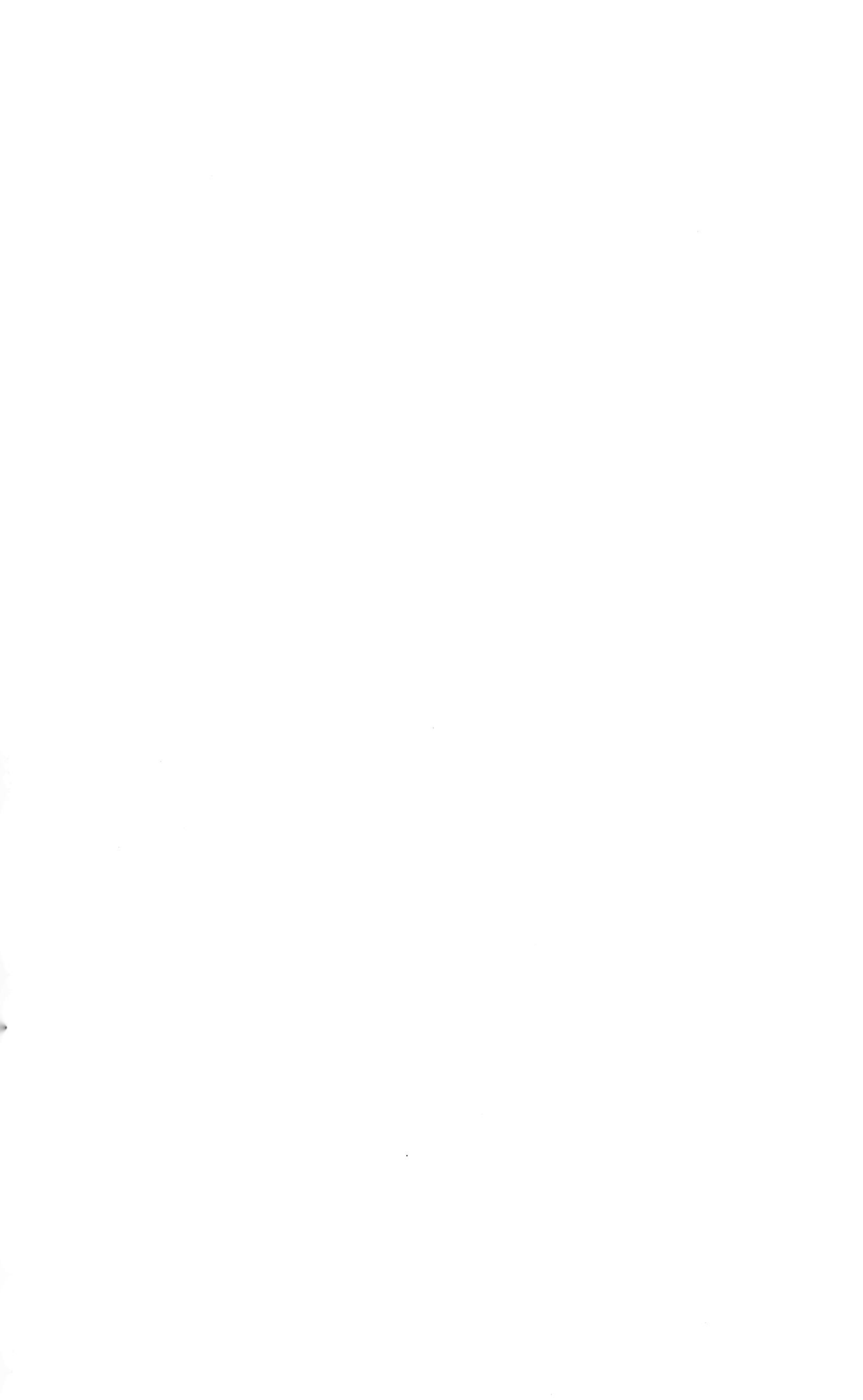

Printed in Great Britain
by Amazon